HONEY

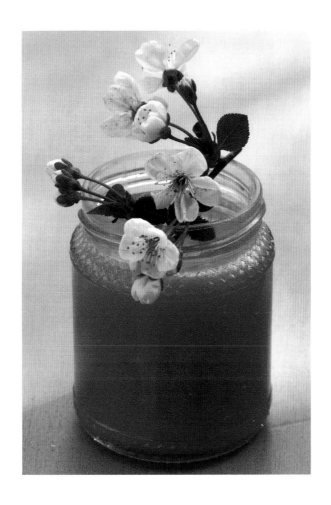

HONEY

NATURE'S WONDER INGREDIENT: 100 AMAZING USES FROM TRADITIONAL
CURES TO FOOD AND BEAUTY, WITH TIPS, HINTS AND 40 TEMPTING RECIPES

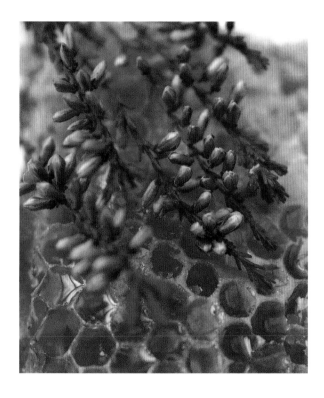

JENNI FLEETWOOD

with photographs by Michelle Garrett

HERMES
HOUSE

This edition is published by Hermes House, an imprint of Anness Publishing Ltd, Hermes House
88–89 Blackfriars Road
London SE1 8HA;
tel. 020 7401 2077; fax 020 7633 9499

www.hermeshouse.com;
www.annesspublishing.com

If you like the images in this book and would like to investigate using them for publishing, promotions or advertising, please visit our website www.practicalpictures.com for more information.

Publisher: Joanna Lorenz
Project Editor: Anne Hildyard
Photography and styling: Michelle Garrett
Designer: Sarah Rock
Contributing Author: Wendy Kavanagh
Production Controller: Wendy Lawson

ETHICAL TRADING POLICY
At Anness Publishing we believe that business should be conducted in an ethical and ecologically sustainable way, with respect for the environment and a proper regard to the replacement of the natural resources we employ.

As a publisher, we use a lot of wood pulp to make high-quality paper for printing, and that wood commonly comes from spruce trees. We are therefore currently growing more than 750,000 trees in three Scottish forest plantations: Berrymoss (130 hectares/320 acres), West Touxhill (125 hectares/305 acres) and Deveron Forest (75 hectares/185 acres). The forests we manage contain more than 3.5 times the number of trees employed each year in making paper for the books we manufacture.

Because of this ongoing ecological investment programme, you, as our customer, can have the pleasure and reassurance of knowing that a tree is being cultivated on your behalf to naturally replace the materials used to make the book you are holding.

Our forestry programme is run in accordance with the UK Woodland Assurance Scheme (UKWAS) and will be certified by the internationally recognized Forest Stewardship Council (FSC). The FSC is a non-government organization dedicated to promoting responsible management of the world's forests. Certification ensures forests are managed in an environmentally sustainable and socially responsible way. For further information about this scheme, go to www.annesspublishing.com/trees

NOTES
Bracketed terms are intended for American readers.

For all recipes, quantities are given in both metric and imperial measures and, where appropriate, in standard cups and spoons. Follow one set of measures, but not a mixture, because they are not interchangeable.

Standard spoon and cup measures are level. 1 tsp = 5ml, 1 tbsp = 15ml, 1 cup = 250ml/8fl oz.

Australian standard tablespoons are 20ml. Australian readers should use 3 tsp in place of 1 tbsp for measuring small quantities.

American pints are 16fl oz/2 cups. American readers should use 20fl oz/2.5 cups in place of 1 pint when measuring liquids.

Electric oven temperatures in this book are for conventional ovens. When using a fan oven, the temperature will probably need to be reduced by about 10–20°C/20–40°F. Since ovens vary, you should check with your manufacturer's instruction book for guidance.

The nutritional analysis given for each recipe is calculated per portion (i.e. serving or item), unless otherwise stated. If the recipe gives a range, such as Serves 4–6, then the nutritional analysis will be for the smaller portion size, i.e. 6 servings. The analysis does not include optional ingredients, such as salt added to taste..

Medium (US large) eggs are used unless otherwise stated.

PUBLISHER'S NOTE
While every effort has been made to ensure accuracy when researching this book, the information on the therapeutic and cosmetic value of honey is often anecdotal and is not intended as a substitute for the advice of a qualified professional. Any use to which the recommendations, ideas and techniques are put is at the reader's sole discretion and risk.

Honey should not be given to children under the age of 1 year. In rare instances, it may contain spores of the bacteria *Clostridium botulinum*. Most older children and adults can cope with this, but because a baby's digestive system is immature, the bacteria can multiply in it and cause problems. If you are pregnant, breastfeeding or have a medical condition and are unsure as to whether you should be having honey, consult your doctor.

The very young, the elderly, pregnant women and those in ill-health or with a compromised immune system are advised against eating dishes containing raw eggs.

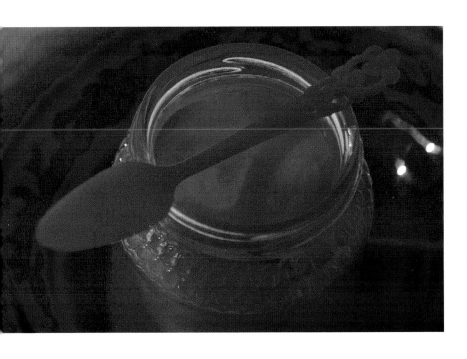
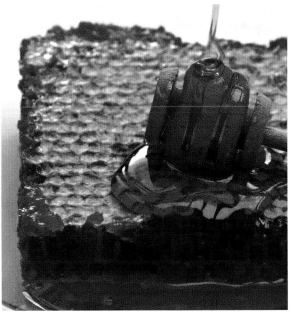

Contents

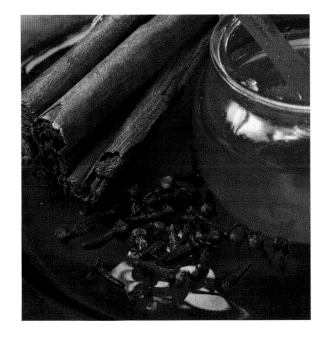
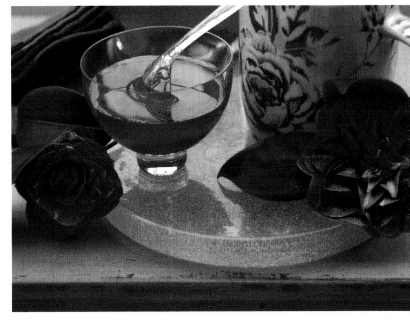

INTRODUCTION

Honey is one of the oldest foods in existence. It has been used for thousands of years in natural remedies and beauty products and in food and drink.

It has been called liquid gold, the golden elixir and the gift of the gods. For centuries, man has harvested honey, revelling in its satisfying sweetness and marvelling at its therapeutic qualities. Globally, honey consumption is at an all-time high, so what better time to examine its benefits and celebrate this remarkable ingredient?

The history of honey is much, much older than mankind. Until recently it was assumed that the bees responsible for this bounty evolved around 60 million years ago. That was until an extraordinary discovery in 2006 – a tiny primitive bee, perfectly preserved in amber, which scientists dated as more than 100 million years old. The find, made in a mine in northern Burma, excited particular interest since the insect had characteristics of both modern bees and wasps, though it favoured the former. This suggests that both types of insect shared a common ancestor.

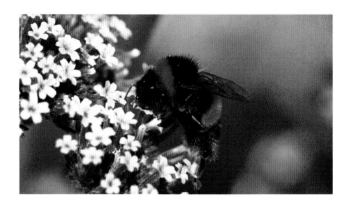

Above: A worker bee gathers pollen and nectar and in the process pollinates the flowers that it visits.

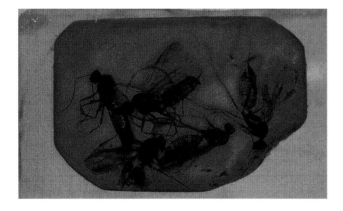

Above: These bees are perfectly preserved in a resin called amber. They are believed to be more than 100 million years old, confirming that bees originated before humans.

Quite when man first stumbled upon honey is not known. Perhaps it was a lucky discovery made when a hunter climbed a tree to escape a wild beast and came across a hive dripping with honey. However it happened, it was the beginning of a love affair with honey that has lasted centuries.

In ancient cultures honey had a role in weddings, births and funerals and in some countries; such as ancient Greece, honey symbolized fertility, beauty and love. Taxes were paid with honey in ancient Egypt and offered to the gods in the form of

a fermented drink that was called 'the nectar of the gods.' As well as its use in the kitchen in food and drink, honey is prized for its healing properties and it is recognized to have antiseptic and antibacterial properties, which can be exploited in natural remedies for various complaints. Honey has the ability to attract and retain moisture, so has a long tradition of being used in creams and lotions. Another useful domestic by-product from the hive is beeswax, which is used to make polishes, soaps, face creams, good quality candles and, with honey, to make lip balms and bath and beauty products.

Considering the astonishing effort that bees make to produce our honey, it is only fitting that the fruit of their labours should be used for so many benefits – adding unique flavour to food, healing remedies, beauty care and some household uses. And it is a totally pure and natural product.

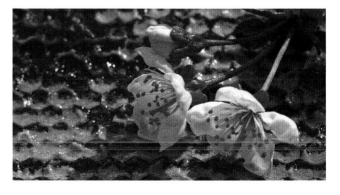

Above: A honeycomb, sealed with wax, contains liquid honey.
Right: The colour of honey varies depending on the floral source.

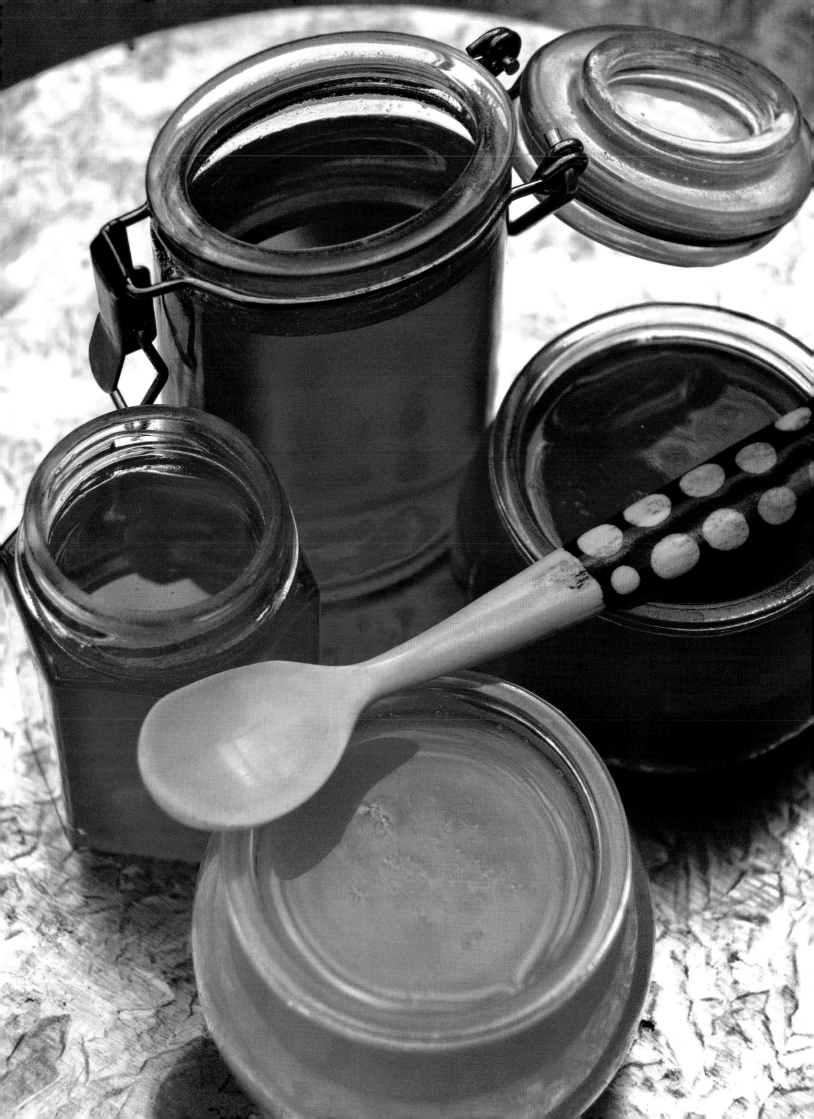

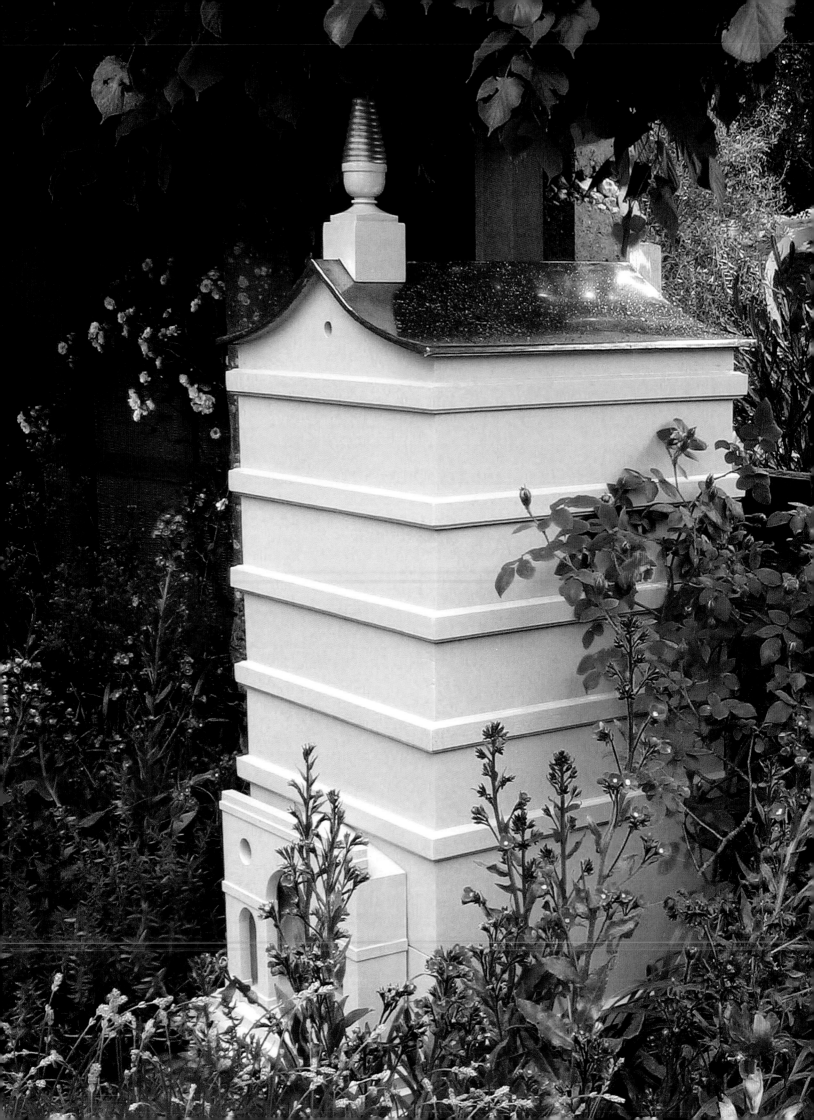

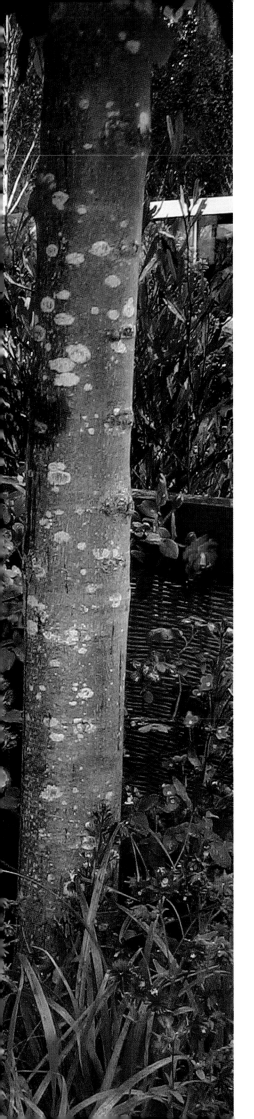

ALL ABOUT HONEY

It is known that primitive people collected and ate wild honey as far back as 7000BCE and ever since, humans have been fascinated by everything related to honey. This chapter explores a selection of superstitions and myths that have grown up around honey. It also explains what honey is; how it is collected and has been over the centuries; and how the beekeeper uses his expertise to help to make different types of honey. The useful by-products of the hive – pollen, propolis, royal jelly and beeswax – are also described.

Left: A beehive is set in a garden with a profusion of colourful flowers.
Foraging bees are attracted to the plants when gathering nectar.

HONEY LEGENDS AND MYTHS

The magical sweetness of honey and its insect origin has made it the subject of enduring myths and legends. Bees, too, have often been used as symbols of the gods.

For centuries, honey has been surrounded by mystique. To the ancients, it seemed inconceivable that so miraculous a substance could actually be produced by insects. Instead, they reasoned that bees must be messengers of the gods, put on Earth to harvest the sweetness that was supplied by divine forces. Honey fell as rain or dew, or was conveyed to Earth by bees that, being magical themselves, were able to flit between heaven and man's domain.

The ancient Egyptians believed that bees were formed from the teardrops of Ra, the Sun God, and honey was his gift to mankind. At one time, Lower Egypt was called Bee Land and the winged insect was a potent symbol.

The association of honey with sunshine and the dawn is also an ancient Indo-Aryan belief. The *Rig-Veda*, Sanskrit scriptures written more than three thousand years ago, ascribe the daily rising of the sun to the Aswins, children of the Sun and Moon, who ride the heavens in a golden chariot filled with honey. Bees and honey have great significance in this sacred work, and incarnations of the gods are often indicated by the presence of bees in religious pictures, sculptures or carvings.

Classical legends

Greek and Roman gods were often associated with bees and honey. Legend has it that the infant Zeus was saved from death by a diet of milk and honey brought by the nymph Melissa after his mother hid him to prevent his father devouring him. But Melissa's role in the

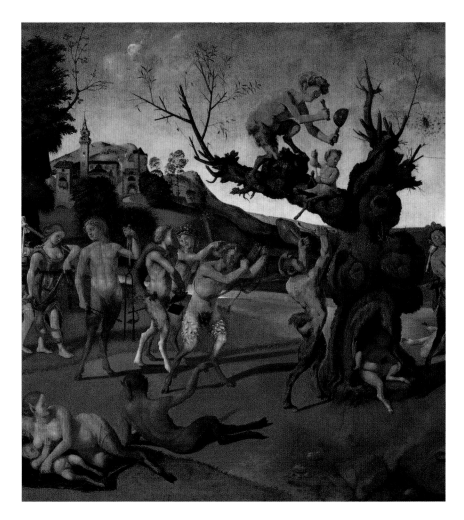

Above: The Discovery of Honey by Bacchus, *c.1499 (tempera on panel) by Piero di Cosimo (c.1642–1521). The scene was described by Ovid in* The Fasti.

deception was discovered, and she was turned into a worm. When Zeus discovered this he was furious, and immediately transformed Melissa into a queen bee, with more bees as attendants.

Ambrosia, the food of the gods, was based on nectar or honey. Honey was believed to come from paradise, and, like the ancient Egyptians, the Greeks believed it dropped from the skies as dew. The Greek historian Plutarch called honey 'the saliva of the stars'.

Many cultures linked stars with bees and honey. Teutonic tribespeople imagined the stars to be swarms of bees, while the moon was a giant bowl, filled with honey and mead. At night it dripped sweetness on to the Earth.

Honey often features in Norse mythology. Mead, an alcoholic drink made from honey, was regularly drunk by Odin and his henchmen, either from their drinking horns or, after battle, from the skulls of their enemies.

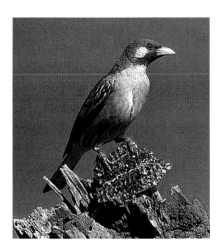

Above: Honey guides feed on bees as they exit the nest, and help people find honey.

African tales

The San people of South Africa and Botswana are often aided in their hunts for wild honey by a honey guide. This is a small bird that likes to feed on bee larvae and beeswax, which it cannot retrieve unaided. The bird therefore enlists the help of either an animal, usually a honey badger, or a human, and attracts attention by making a shrill cry and fluttering until its elected assistant begins to follow. It then heads for the bees' nest, stopping and waiting several times if necessary, until it is certain that it is being followed.

The San always leave a generous portion of honeycomb for the bird, for if they fail to do so, they believe that next time the honey guide appears, it will lead them straight toward a leopard or a venomous snake.

In West Africa and Cuba, honey is associated with the Yoruba goddess of love, Oshun, who is always depicted wearing a yellow dress. Oshun is a water spirit, symbolizing clarity. She is also linked to fertility and childbearing. Women who ask her help bring her offerings of honey, which they first taste to ensure it has not been tampered with by someone who wishes the goddess ill.

Superstitions

Many cultures believe bees to be the souls of the dead. There is a superstition that they must always be informed of important events in the family, especially if there is a death. In parts of the United States, if a beekeeper dies, the new keeper must tell the bees what has happened, and inform them that he is now their master.

Bees must be informed of weddings, too, and should be told if they are about to be moved. If a bee flies into your house, you can expect a visitor, and if the bee circles a sleeping child, the infant will be blessed with good luck and long life. Nobody knows the precise origin of the word honeymoon but it may go back to the days of the ancient Egyptians, when honey was used in marriage rituals. In medieval Europe, newlyweds were given enough mead to last them from one full moon to the next. This may explain how the word came to be used after a wedding. In Anglo-Saxon England, the bride's father supplied the mead, which was believed to enhance fertility.

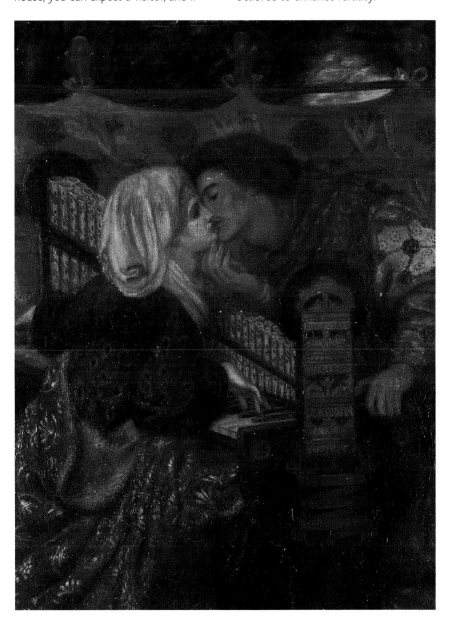

Above: This picture by Rossetti, c.1850, is of Rene D'Anjou and Jeanne de Laval enjoying their honeymoon. It may be a myth, but it is thought honey was used in marriage rites.

WHAT IS HONEY?

Honey undergoes a complex process in the hive to convert it from nectar to a golden liquid. Moisture is removed, then the honeycomb cells are sealed with wax to protect the honey.

To understand what honey is, it is first necessary to know a little about nectar, a sweet liquid produced by plants to attract female worker bees and other insects to the flowers, and thus assist in the process of pollination. When a bee lands on a flower it is guided to the nectar by a pattern of lines on the petals. These marks, or nectar guides, are difficult for a human to detect, but they are specifically tailored to a bee's vision and act like signposts for bees.

Nectar is a solution of sugars in water, with small amounts of amino acids, vitamins, proteins and enzymes. The precise chemical composition and concentration varies, depending on the type of plant, the soil in which it grows, temperature and humidity levels and moisture in the soil. Bees tend not to mix sources when on a foraging flight, but collect all their nectar from one type of plant. This pattern of behaviour is exploited by beekeepers intent on producing monofloral honeys (from a single source). When the chosen flower comes into bud, they make sure that the supers (boxes above the brood boxes in which the bees store honey) in their hives are completely drained of the last type of honey produced. With their favourite food within reach, the bees will confine themselves to the source selected for them by the beekeeper.

Honeybees

There are around 20,000 species of bees. Most species are solitary, and while they collect nectar and pollen, they do this purely for their own use. Only a few

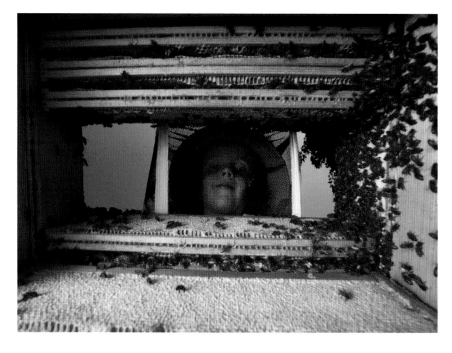

Above: A little boy looks through the viewing panel in a beehive to check out what is happening inside the hive. This facility helps beekeepers spot any infestations in the hive.

varieties of bees store honey. These include the South American stingless bees and bumblebees. For champion honey production, however, no bee is as efficient as the true honeybee. There are several types of honeybees, including dwarf and giant species. All live in complex colonies, but many are not suitable for containment in hives. The domesticated bee is *Apis mellifera*. Native to Europe, Africa and the Middle East, this type of bee now has a huge range, since it has been introduced into North and South America, and Australia.

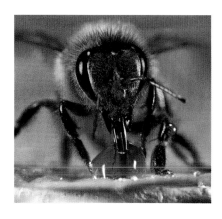

Above: This magnified picture shows a honeybee sucking up nectar.

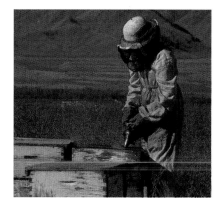

Above: A beekeeper in Utah uses smoke to calm bees before moving the hive.

From nectar to honey

The conversion of nectar to honey begins while the bee is still in flight. Various enzymes are added to the nectar, the most notable of which is invertase. This breaks down sucrose in the nectar into glucose and fructose.

Back at the hive, the bee regurgitates the partially processed nectar and transfers it to waiting worker bees. They work it in their mouths, adding more enzymes before depositing the sap in an empty cell in the brood box.

For the processed nectar to be transformed into honey, about half of its moisture content must be removed. This happens in two ways: by evaporation, due to the heat inside the hive, and by fanning, a process whereby worker bees waft warm air over the cells. As the moisture level decreases and the solution becomes more concentrated, more chemical changes occur in the sap.

When a cell is almost full to the brim, and the moisture content has dropped to 18 per cent, the cells are sealed with wax to prevent further moisture loss and protect the contents.

Composition of honey

The composition of individual types of honey varies considerably. All honey is primarily a highly concentrated sugar solution. The main sugars in honey (about 85 per cent of the solids present) are fructose and glucose, which are both simple sugars, but there will also be small amounts of as many as 22 complex sugars, including sucrose.

In general, there will be slightly more fructose than glucose, making the honey less likely to crystallize. Acacia honey is very resistant to crystallization, due to its high fructose levels. Rapeseed, or canola, honey, in which glucose is dominant, granulates very quickly.

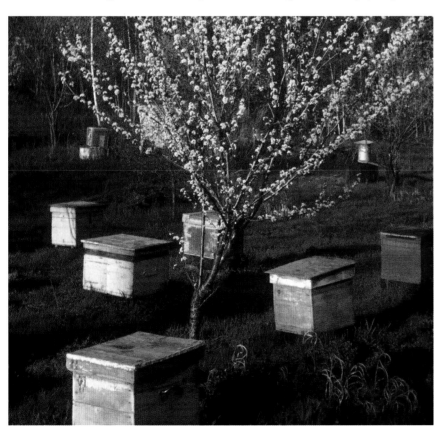

Above: Hives are arranged around fruit trees in Siberia, Russia. Bees and other insects visit the blossoms to gather nectar and to assist in pollination.

BEES AT RISK

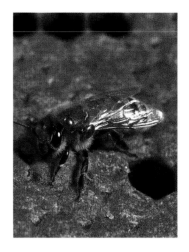

*Above: An adult worker bee has been infected by two parasitic mites (*Varroa destructor*) on its thorax.*

For many years beekeepers have worried about dwindling stocks. In the United States alone, it has been estimated that the number of managed bees in hives has declined by up to a quarter. Wild bees are also affected.

The phenomenon is causing great concern, not just because of what it means in terms of honey production, but also because of its effect on the pollination of plants and therefore food stocks.

A number of reasons have been suggested for the decline in bee populations. Most of the blame has been directed at parasites and diseases. Mites such as *Varroa destructor* and *Acarapis woodi* caused major losses in the 1980s and 90s, and foul brood disease has been a widespread problem.

The use of pesticides has killed bees in large numbers. Loss of habitat is another issue. Modern farming methods often devote huge swathes of land to a single crop. When it flowers, there is ample food for the bees, but when the nectar flow is over, they are in serious trouble. Many beekeepers address this problem by moving the hives but this can stress the bees and spread infection.

Colony Collapse Disorder, in which formerly healthy hives are discovered to be almost empty, is a huge concern. Experts are unsure as to the cause of the collapse.

BEEKEEPING THROUGH THE AGES

The development of beekeeping took honey from being an occasional treat to a useful source of sweetness that could be easily harvested from tailor-made hives.

Apiculture, or beekeeping, probably began around 3000 to 4000BC. The first beekeepers, as opposed to hunters, simply searched for a hollow tree in which wild bees had made their nest. They cut down the tree, isolated the portion of trunk containing the nest, and carried this home. When it was realized that bees would be equally happy in man-made objects, provided these were dark, dry and defensible, swarms of bees were encouraged to occupy these instead. Some cultures used vertical, hollow pipes made from wood or clay as rudimentary hives; others employed clay or pottery urns or constructed containers from cork or reeds.

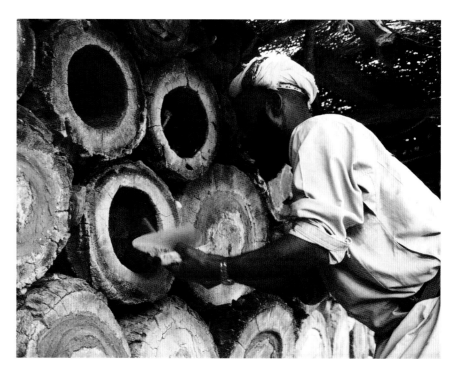

Above: A beekeeper carefully removes honey from a beehive. In the Oman, beehives are not conventional designs, but are often made from stacked, hollow palm tree trunks.

Beekeeping in Egypt and Mesopotamia

Inscriptions on Sumerian tablets suggest that they were among the world's first beekeepers, but it was the ancient Egyptians who really developed the craft. Wild swarms were enticed into specially constructed pottery containers, which were then taken back to the temples and given into the care of priests. By 2600BC apiculture was well established and honey was used medicinally, in beauty preparations and for trade, 110 pots of honey being equal in value to an ox or an ass.

The symbol for honey in Egyptian hieroglyphics was a bee, and beekeeping was represented on reliefs in the Temple of the Sun at Abusir. These carvings show honey being transferred from clay hives to containers for storage. The ancient Egyptians also practised migratory beekeeping, loading the hives on to rafts that were moved along the Nile so that the bees could gather nectar from plants as they came into full flower. When the nectar ceased to flow, in early February, the itinerant beekeepers returned to Cairo and sold their honey in the markets there.

The ancient Egyptians liked to use honey in cooking, especially for honey cakes, and as offerings to the gods. Jars of honey were buried with the pharaohs, to sustain them in the afterlife, a practice that was also common in Mesopotamia (modern day Iraq), where honey was widely used medicinally.

There are many references to honey in the Bible and it is known that ancient Palestine was a good source of wild honey. In India, too, the use of honey was widespread. It played (and continues to play) an important role in Ayurvedic medicine, a system of healthcare based on Sanskrit texts that are believed to be more than 3000 years old.

Beekeeping in Greece and Rome

From Egypt, beekeeping spread to ancient Greece and Rome. Aristotle, Hippocrates and Dioscorides sang honey's praises, variously recommending it as a wound salve, a cough medicine, an aid to eliminating body lice, and a cure for earache, ulcers and even haemorrhoids. In Greek mythology there are references to honey, which was regarded as the food of the gods. It was the Greeks who first fully appreciated the subtle differences in flavour in honeys from different sources. Savory and marjoram got honourable mention, but in the opinion of the Greeks the finest honey came from thyme, especially thyme growing on the slopes of Mount Hymettus, near Athens. Honey was the only sweetener available in Europe at the time, aside from syrups made from dried fruits, and herbs such as sweet cicely. It was also widely used for making mead, or honey wine.

The ancient Romans valued honey as much as the Greeks. Apicius, a famous gourmand writing in the 1st century BC, extolled its virtues, using honey in more than half of his recipes, including one for roast dormouse (brushed with honey) and another for honey-baked ham. Honey was often mixed with salty ingredients such as anchovies to create sweet-sour sauces. It was also highly valued as a food preservative.

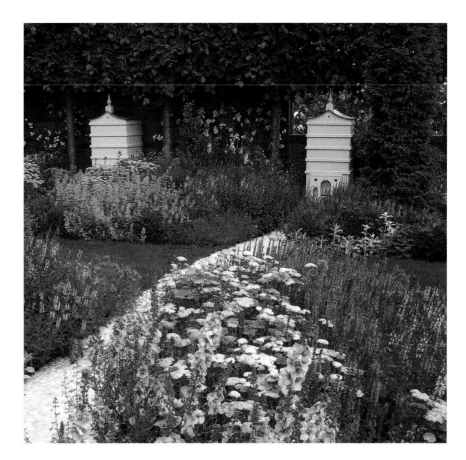

Above: Two modern beehives are set in a garden with a profusion of colourful flowers. Foraging worker bees are attracted to a wide variety of plants when gathering nectar.

Beekeeping in Britain

How and when beekeeping reached the British Isles isn't known precisely. There is evidence that wild bees were exploited from the very earliest times. Traces of honey have been found on Neolithic pottery remains dating from around five thousand years ago, and beekeeping was apparently practised in England long before the Roman invasion. By the 11th century AD, beekeeping was widespread and was so important that the Domesday Book lists the number of hives each land holder possessed. The hives were often made of wicker, and sometimes they were covered with tree bark or clay.

Skeps, or bee baskets, consisted of coils of straw, reed or grass, bound with hazel or willow fronds. Over decades, hives became more sophisticated and beekeepers tried a variety of different sizes and shapes. Some hives had glass windows inserted in the walls so that people could watch the bees inside; some were placed inside sturdier containers for protection; others were raised on stones to make them less accessible to mice and rats.

Beekeeping and the collection and preparation of honey and beeswax, traditionally male pursuits, later became the province of the woman of the house.

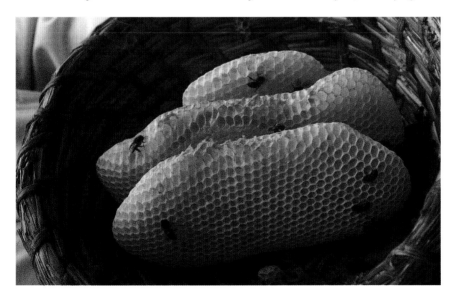

Above: These straw skeps or bee baskets look attractive but it is far easier to look after bees in hives, and also removing honey from a skep can be damaging.

THE PRODUCTION OF HONEY

Beekeepers manage millions of colonies of bees around the world. Together, they produce 300 million pounds of honey each year, in a variety of forms and flavours.

There are thousands of different types of honey. Since bees will take nectar from any flowering plant, the range is almost infinite. Although honey is produced commercially on a grand scale, it can be hugely rewarding to get to know local beekeepers who can tell you which plants are likely to have provided the nectar for the honey they sell, and who may well offer different types of honey at different stages of the season.

Regulations govern the sale of honey and help to ensure that what is on sale is, as the definition states, a 100 per cent natural product. Honey may not have sugar or starch added to it, and there are strict rules governing colour, blend and composition.

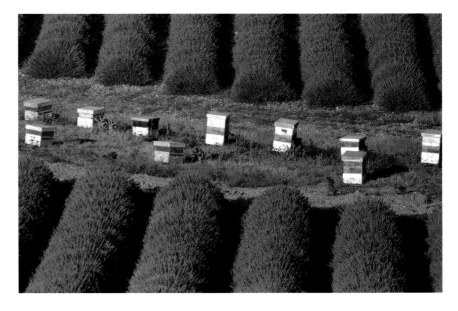

Above: The beautiful violet flowers of lavender attract bees because of their colour and perfume. Nectar from lavender produces honey with a distinctive flavour.

Source of nectar
Most honey is polyfloral, which means that it is made from the nectar of a variety of flowers. Although on each collecting foray a bee will gather nectar from only one type of plant, on subsequent trips she may well visit other flowers, so the honey harvested from the hive will ultimately come from several sources.

However, if there is a local abundance of a particular type of flowering plant which the bees favour, or if bee hives are taken to fields where only one type of plant is cultivated, the chances are that the honey produced will be monofloral, or predominantly from a single source. The third category is blended honey, where different varieties (sometimes from different countries) will be carefully mixed to provide a consistent flavour and colour.

The waggle dance
Scout bees are bees that convey information about a desirable nectar and pollen source to forager bees. This is known as the waggle dance and it is always done on the face of the honeycomb. The display is very distinctive and follows a figure-of-eight pattern. The direction in which the scout

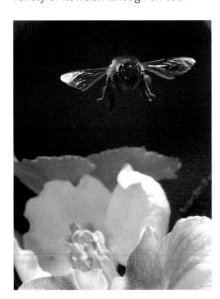

Above: A bee collecting nectar hovers over apple blossom.

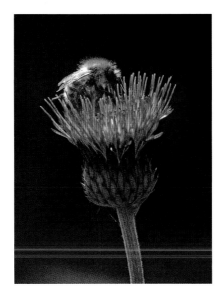

Above: A bee sucks up nectar from clover to produce a popular honey.

bee moves, relative to the position of the sun, gives the foragers information about the route they need to follow. How lively the scout is, and how loudly she buzzes, apparently conveys more detail, such as the distance to the flowers. Finally, the perfume from the pollen she has collected at the site suggests which type of flowering plant is providing the provender for that day.

Colour

Most honey is golden in colour. Hold it up to the light and it looks like bottled sunshine. However, honey can be so pale as to be almost white or so dark as to rival mahogany. The variations depend on the plant source, although some changes in colour can occur during processing or storage. Paler honey sells better than dark honey. However, as consumers become more aware of the many different varieties of honey on the

market, darker honeys are becoming more popular. Aside from more pronounced flavours, dark honeys have more antioxidants than pale ones.

In addition to the colours listed above, there have been instances where bees have produced pink, green or even blue honey. Unusual colours are often the result of an accident. Discarded confectionery boxes draw bees, and if the sugar in the box is brightly coloured, the honey will be too. In rare instances, an unusual colour can be a natural phenomenon. In the American state of North Carolina, honey may be blue. Locals attribute this to huckleberries, but no one is sure what causes the effect.

Aroma and flavour

Not all honeys smell the same. Some, especially those based on citrus, have a distinctive scent that intensifies when the honey is warmed. Open a jar of orange blossom honey that has been standing on a breakfast table in the garden on a sunny morning and the perfume will be irresistible. Honey connoisseurs, like professional wine tasters, pay much attention to the 'nose'.

The flavour of honey is determined by the plant nectar from which it came. If the honey is polyfloral, someone with an educated palate may be able to detect the dominant source, at least, but the flavour is not likely to be particularly noteworthy. Where bees forage among mixed plants, as in a wild flower meadow, each batch of honey may be slightly different, depending on the proportions of the various nectars. This is part of the magic if you are buying honey from a small independent producer, but in the commercial world blending will almost certainly have ironed out these subtle differences.

Like the colour, the flavour of honey varies enormously. It can be bland,

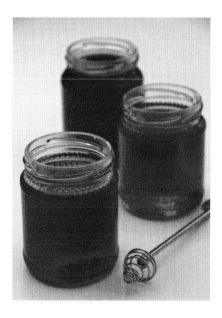

Above: Despite the belief that honey is golden in colour, there are numerous shades of honey; these are just three examples of different hues.

subtle, scented, sweet, bitter – even brash. At honey tastings, individuals are blindfolded and then invited to try a selection of honeys. Most novices are amazed to discover how much the flavours vary. Some honeys make an immediate impact. Others are more subtle, but with flavours that develop in the mouth. One or two varieties have a definite aftertaste. There are hundreds of types of honey to choose from, sourced from many different countries, and what one person likes, another may loathe. People who don't like honey may not have tasted enough varieties.

Consistency

Honey can be naturally thin or thick. The moisture content varies a lot. Some types seldom crystallize; others solidify so rapidly that the honey is extremely difficult to extract. A few honeys are thixotropic, which means that they are gel-like in the jar but liquefy if shaken. For many people, texture – the way the honey feels in the mouth – is an important part of the tasting experience.

LOCATION

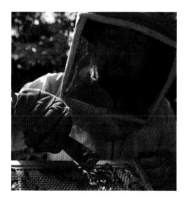

Honey is produced in countries all over the world, from Siberia to the tip of South America. In many countries, the demand for honey outstrips local supply, so that supplies have to be imported. Of the many factors affecting honey production, weather is paramount. Where the climate is hot all year round, as in equatorial regions, the production of honey is more or less continuous. In colder climates, if the temperature drops too much the bees will die.

POLLEN, PROPOLIS AND ROYAL JELLY

Honey is not the only valuable product produced by bees. Pollen, propolis and royal jelly are used for food or building purposes in the hive, and they are used therapeutically by humans.

Pollen

In addition to collecting nectar to turn into honey, bees forage for pollen, mixing it with saliva and nectar and bringing it back to the hive in the form of neat pellets, which they pack in 'pollen baskets' on their hind legs. The pellets are deposited in storage cells and turned into 'bee bread' by worker bees or collected by the beekeeper; the bees squeeze through a small gap in the hive and the pollen is scraped off their legs as they enter. After the first three days of life, the larvae of all bees other than the queen are fed on this nutritious compound. Pollen is sometimes used as a food supplement, but there are some questions over its efficacy. Side effects have been reported.

Propolis

Bees make propolis, which is incredibly sticky, from resins, saps and other substances that they gather from trees and plants. It is basically a mixture of resin, balm and wax, with essential oils, pollen, organic substances and minerals.

There's rather more evidence of the positive effects of propolis than there is for bee pollen. Propolis is the cement-like substance bees use both when building – to fill holes, reinforce combs and repair damaged cells – and as a disinfectant. The word propolis was allegedly coined by Aristotle. It means 'on behalf of the city' and Aristotle felt it was an apt description of a substance that has many uses in strengthening the hive and keeping it hygienic. A hive

HONEYDEW

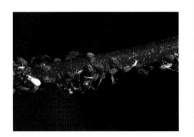

Not all honey comes from nectar. A small proportion is made from honeydew, a liquid that is secreted by aphids and other similar insects. This syrupy substance has a sweet taste, like nectar, and bees will sometimes harvest it. Honeydew honey is similar to nectar honey but doesn't contain pollen. In some parts of the world, honeydew honey is highly valued, but some claim that it is often contaminated with environmental pollutants and mould spores.

containing upwards of 50,000 bees in temperatures of around 35°C/95°F and 90 per cent humidity would seem to be the ideal breeding ground for bacteria, yet because bees polish every surface with propolis, infection occurs much less frequently than one might expect.

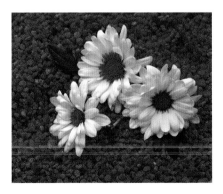

Above: Pollen grains, which are gathered at the entrance to the beehive.

Above: This artificially coloured electron micrograph of pollen grains shows the sculpted surfaces that allow them to catch the wind and pollinate a female flower.

Propolis is also used to line cells before the queen lays her eggs, again creating a sterile environment.

It is claimed that propolis can alleviate painful joints, treat eczema, relieve respiratory conditions, heal wounds and burns and treat gastro-intestinal problems. It also stimulates the immune system. Many beekeepers simply scrape it off the interior of their hives and take a little every day in alcohol. Health food shops sell propolis in tablet form or as a liquid or spray. Diluted in warm water and used as a gargle, it is said to offer protection against colds and flu. Propolis is also used medicinally to combat gingivitis. Some studies into propolis and royal jelly have suggested that these products may have some value in restricting the growth of certain malignant tumours, but the research is still in its infancy.

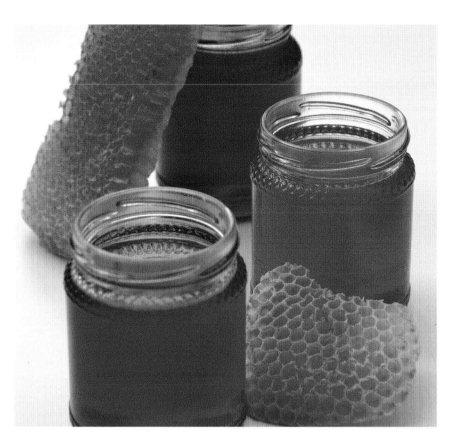

Above: Clear honeys in different colours and beautifully constructed honeycomb are the fruits of the bees' labour. One jar of honey is made of nectar from millions of flowers.

Royal jelly

Quite why a diet of royal jelly turns a regular bee grub into a queen is not fully understood. This creamy substance, produced in the hypopharyngeal glands of worker bees, is fed to all larvae for a few days when they first hatch.

When a hive needs a new queen, several larvae are chosen. Instead of being weaned on to bee bread, they are initially fed royal jelly, then they will eat honey and pollen. One of these larvae will become the new queen and she will continue to dine only on royal jelly for the rest of her life. The queen can choose whether or not to fertilize the egg she lays; drones (male bees that have no sting and do not collect nectar) come from unfertilized eggs, while the females such as worker bees and queens come from fertilized eggs. Queens live for years, unlike worker bees and drones, whose lifespans are counted in weeks.

Young workers feed the larvae, clean the hive and produce royal jelly until the glands fail and they then start to build the honeycomb. They then leave the hive and work as a forager.

The link between longevity of the queeen bee and royal jelly has led to the latter being endowed with mystical qualities. Extravagant claims are made for royal jelly but these appear to have little foundation in fact.

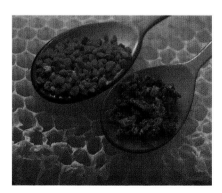

Above: Pollen (left) and propolis (right) are both used as food supplements.

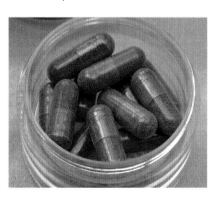

Above: Propolis is available in health food shops in capsule form.

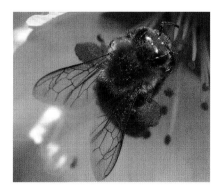

Above: The orange-yellow pollen baskets can be clearly seen on the bee's legs.

HONEYCOMBS AND BEESWAX

Beeswax honeycombs are wonderful feats of engineering. The perfectly formed hexagons are the strongest and smallest possible shapes in which to store the maximum amount of honey.

Although everyone is familiar with honey, another product that the industrious bee makes is the lesser known, but no less useful, beeswax. The production of beeswax is essential to the bee colony. They raise their young in the wax comb and use it as storage for surplus honey for the winter.

Beeswax is produced by young worker bees after they have eaten large quantities of honey or sugar syrup. The bees gather together, which raises their temperature and they begin to 'sweat.' The heat that is generated stimulates the production of beeswax, which is formed by wax-producing glands as small, thin scales or flakes on the underside of the bees' abdomen. Other worker bees gather the wax scales and use it to make sheets of hexagonal shaped cells or they transfer the wax scales to the part of the hive that needs some new wax to repair damaged cells.

Beeswax in the hive

There is a very low yield of beeswax. Young worker bees that are between 12 and 17 days old produce the beeswax. What is remarkable is that bees need to eat ten parts of honey to produce one part of beeswax, and it is estimated that bees must fly around 150,000 miles (530,000 kilometres) to produce just one pound (450g) of beeswax. Additionally, the size of the wax glands depends on the age of the worker bee.

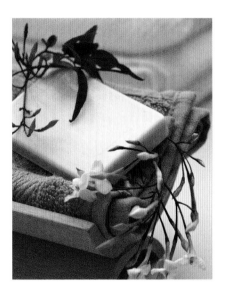

Above: Soap made from beeswax has good moisturizing qualities.

The wax glands eventually start to atrophy after the worker bee has made many daily flights.

Beekeepers regularly remove wax from the hive; this encourages the bees to build new wax combs. The wax that is produced is at first white, but owing to the influence of pollen and propolis, it gradually changes to a yellow or brown colour. It is perfectly safe to eat, as are the cappings with which the bees seal the honey cells. Wax that has been used for rearing the new brood is usually dirty and contaminated and is discarded. The wax in which the bees store the honey is fairly clean and can be melted down, filtered and sold.

Temperature control

Beeswax has to be at just the right temperature to allow the bees to mould it into the correct shape. If the temperature is too low, the beeswax

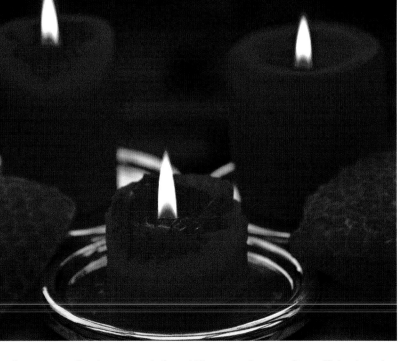

Above: Beeswax candles that are made from 100 per cent beeswax burn efficiently and completely. They do not smoke or drip, and have a pleasant aroma.

will be too brittle and will break up. If the temperature is too high, it will melt. To ensure that they can manipulate the beeswax, the hive is maintained at a temperature of 35°C/95°F.

Varied uses of beeswax

One of the main uses of beeswax is in making high-quality candles, which are used in the home and in churches because they burn hotter, brighter and cleaner than commercial candles. In skin-care products, beeswax has proved to be a superior barrier cream. Its emollient qualities are also recognized in soap making. Some cheeses even have a beeswax coating, which protects the cheese as it ages and does not impart odd flavours.

TIPS FOR MELTING BEESWAX

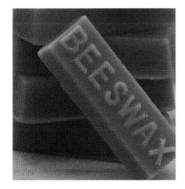

When melting beeswax, the safest way is to use a bain marie – a small saucepan containing the wax that sits inside a larger pan of water. The wax should not be melted in a pan that is directly over a heat source, such as an electric ring or gas flame, since this can damage the beeswax and if it ignites accidentally, it will burn fiercely. Beeswax gets hotter and hotter until it ignites so it should not be close to a heat source.

The best containers in which to melt beeswax are stainless steel or plated pans. Metals such as copper, brass or iron impart colour to the wax and cause it to look dull. Be cautious when you are pouring out hot beeswax as it has the potential to cause serious burns.

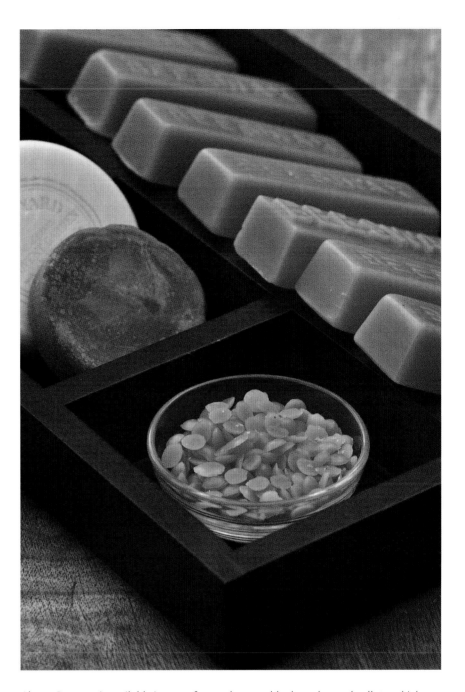

Above: Beeswax is available in many forms: there are blocks, cakes and pellets, which are quicker to melt down when making soaps and candles.

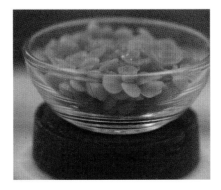

Above: Beeswax pellets are useful when small quantities of wax are required.

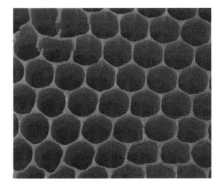

Above: A close up of the six-sided cylinders that make up honeycomb.

DIFFERENT FORMS OF HONEY

There are lots of different ways in which honey is sold. You can choose from fresh honeycomb, cut comb, raw honey, heat-treated honey, set honey or organic honey.

Honeycomb

This is the bees' own packaging system. If offered for sale it must be fresh from the hive, and may not contain any eggs or larvae. Before the advent of the honey extraction machine, this is how most people enjoyed honey, but today it is quite difficult to obtain. Biting into the comb (which is edible) breaks the bees' seals on the honeycomb cells and lets the honey flow into your mouth.

Cut comb or chunk honey

This is liquid honey with pieces of honeycomb added to the jar. Acacia honey, which is mild and light, is often used as the base. Acacia honey remains liquid, showing off the honeycomb.

Raw honey

The natural product that has been drained from a honeycomb after the wax covering on the cells has been removed is called raw honey. It will contain some pollen and wax particles. If pressure is applied in the process it will be described as pressed honey. In commercial terms, honey labelled as raw may only have been subjected to minimum processing and low heat.

Liquid honey

This is the most popular form of honey, and the most versatile. When honey is extracted from the comb, it naturally retains some particles of wax, along with propolis and pollen grains. There is a ready market for the natural product, especially if the honey is to be used medicinally. However, these substances give the honey a slightly cloudy appearance. To counter this, beekeepers filter honey through fine mesh, which removes the wax and propolis but leaves the protein-rich pollen behind. It sells in health food shops and at farmers' markets.

Pasteurized or heat-treated honey

In health and hygiene terms, there is no reason why honey should be pasteurized. Its high sugar content protects against the growth of bacteria, and spores of *Clostridium botulinum*, the bacteria that can spell danger for babies, are not destroyed by heat. Pasteurization is carried out largely to satisfy the requirements of industry, since the honey is then less likely to granulate or ferment even if storage conditions are less than perfect. Supermarkets require packagers to produce a clear product. To achieve this, the honey is heated, then put through a rigorous filtration process. Heating dissolves the 'seed crystals' in the honey so it is less likely to granulate.

Set honey

This term can be applied to any honey that has solidified through crystallization of the sugars it contains. This natural process happens faster in some types of honey than in others, usually when there is a high proportion of glucose. Honey that has crystallized spontaneously is grainy, even gritty, and is difficult to get out of the jar, but it can be liquified if it is warmed gently. Do not let it get too hot, or nutrients will be destroyed.

Creamed honey

Also described as whipped, churned, spun honey or honey fondant, this is honey that has been deliberately crystallized in controlled conditions so

Left: Creamed honey is also varied in colour depending on the floral source.

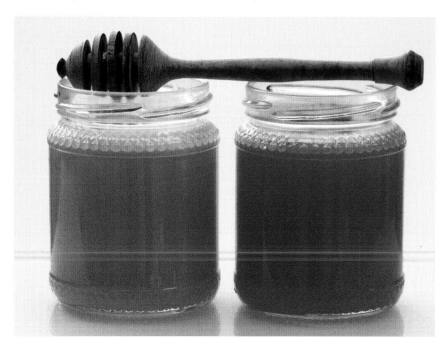

that it forms a smooth mixture. Honey that is high in glucose and will crystallize readily is ideal for creaming. Clover, sunflower and Tasmanian leatherwood are typical examples. The honey is heated, filtered, cooled and chilled. The honey blender 'seeds' the fresh honey with an already crystalline honey of the same type. There is a real art to the operation, since the honey crystals must be kept small and uniform. The mixture is churned, then bottled. At this stage the honey is creamy, setting to a spreading consistency in the jar.

Organic honey

This is subject to strict guidelines. The beehives must be on land that has been certified as organic. Radiating out from the hives, for 6 kilometres/4 miles in any direction, all sources of nectar must be organic crops or untreated wild flowers. The zone may not contain motorways, urban centres, waste dumps or other potential sources of contaminants. Look for a certified product with a label on the jars, stating that the honey comes from approved organic areas.

Honey sticks

These are sold as sweet treats. Slim plastic tubes are filled with pure honey to provide a handy snack or sweetener for tea or coffee.

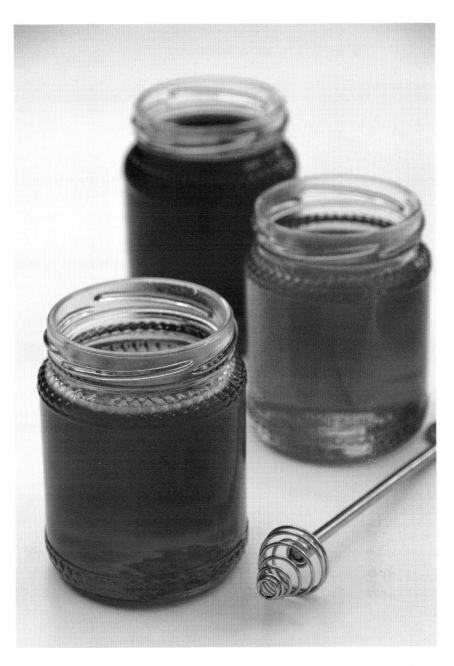

Above: Whether you choose a light or dark honey is really is just a matter of personal preference. Some dark honeys may have a more assertive flavour.

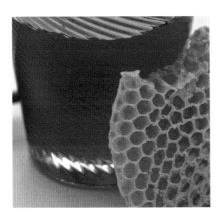

Above: Two different types of honey: clear honey and honeycomb.

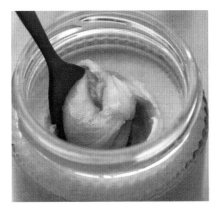

Above: Creamed honey has been whipped to produce a smooth, thick mixture.

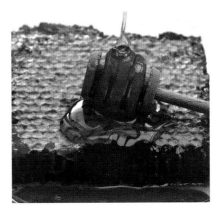

Above: A wooden honey spoon helps to obtain the honey without dripping it.

POPULAR HONEYS

Honey comes in so many textures and flavours that it can be difficult to choose between them. Make the most of tasting opportunities to try something new.

There are many different types of honey on the market, yet most of us seldom search out the specific. We may prefer our honey set or clear, but that's often as far as choosing a honey goes. Others are more particular, and wouldn't dream of simply picking up the first jar they find on the shelf. Although the differences are more subtle, honey is just as varied as jam, so it is well worth experimenting.

Some honey is labelled by the country of origin. Mexican honey, for instance, is a medium-bodied polyfloral honey from the Yucatan region. It has a rich, fruity flavour and strong floral scent. Australian honey, largely from eucalyptus, has a definite toffee flavour with a hint of raisin. It comes mainly from south-eastern Australia, especially Victoria and New South Wales.

Caribbean honey, another polyfloral, has a rich amber colour and robust, fruity flavour that goes well with rum. Chilean honey typically has a fruity flavour with a hint of vanilla. Honey that is simply labelled 'English' will often be based on nectar from wild flowers and hedgerow blossoms. One of the most popular varieties is a creamed honey with a fudge-like flavour. English beekeeper's honey is direct from the hive and has not been processed commercially. Zambian forest honey has excited interest. This creamy, delectable honey comes from bark hives that are hung in the Miombo forests in the north-west of the country.

There are no specific rules requiring the country of origin to be listed on honey labels, but if an indication is given, the honey must originate wholly from that country. If honey is a blend from various geographical sources, the label should make that clear.

The list that follows is intended to introduce the most popular or typical honeys, plus some rarer types. Most are ascribed to a particular plant, although in reality they are all described as monoflorals; that is, the source is the nectar from the blossoms of that single plant, which is then made into honey. The pictures on these pages show a wide range of honeys from different countries, not all of which have text entries.

Acacia honey

This pale yellow honey has a mild, sweet, floral flavour with hints of vanilla. It actually comes from nectar from the false acacia tree, *Robinia pseudoacacia*. Native to the United States, where it is known as the black locust tree, *Robinia pseudoacacia* is widely cultivated in Hungary, Bulgaria, Romania, France and Italy. Slow to crystallize, as a result of its high fructose levels, acacia honey remains liquid for long periods. It is a good honey for cooking, as it mixes easily in liquids, such as drinks or batters. Cut honeycomb is often placed in jars of acacia honey, since its clarity and pale colour allow the comb to be seen to advantage. It is often blended with other types of honey.

Alfalfa honey

Popular in parts of the United States, this very pale, almost white honey has a delicate flavour. It is not particularly sweet, and sometimes has a slight spiciness, which makes it a useful ingredient for dressings and sauces.

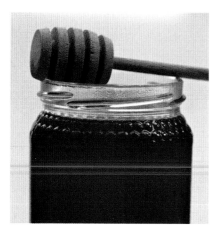

Australian eucalyptus honey

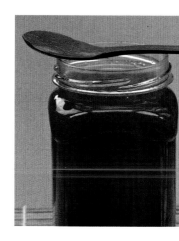

Australian manuka honey

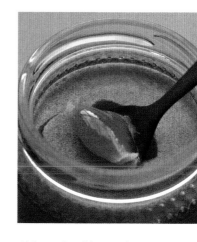

Chilean ulmo blossom honey

Cotswold clear honey

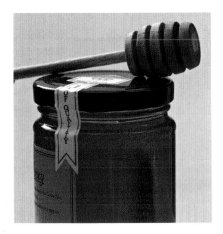

European acacia honey

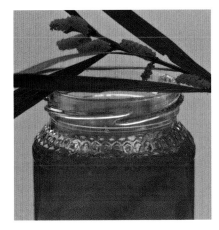

English beekeeper's honey

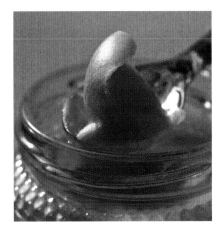

Apple blossom honey

This pale gold honey is produced in the spring. It has a sweet flavour with a hint of apple. Some beekeepers in Kent and the English West Country produce it, either as a monofloral or as a polyfloral with wild flowers. In the United States apple blossom honey comes mainly from states in the north and centre of the country.

Arbutus (strawberry tree) honey

The source of this rare and expensive honey is the strawberry tree, a beautiful evergreen that produces exquisite white flowers in the autumn. Native to south-west Ireland and the Mediterranean, the tree takes its name from the small red fruit that it produces. Arbutus honey is amber in colour, with green and grey tones. It has a pungent aroma and bitter flavour that is very much an acquired taste. Arbutus honey is valued for its therapeutic qualities.

Avocado honey

California and Israel are the main producers of this dark, velvety honey. It tastes nothing like avocado, but has a flavour reminiscent of molasses.

Blackberry honey

This honey is more common in the United States. The colour ranges from white to pale amber. Although brambles or blackberries grow profusely in the United Kingdom, this type of honey is rare there.

Blueberry honey

Popular in the eastern United States and Canada, blueberry honey is said to smell like lemon leaves. It has a fruity flavour, which some claim really does remind them of blueberries, and a delicate, buttery aftertaste. The colour is golden to medium amber.

Borage honey

Bees love the pretty blue flowers of this common plant, and their nectar produces a pale, delicately flavoured honey. Borage is widely grown in the United Kingdom and on the South Island of New Zealand. This type of honey is slow to crystallize. New Zealanders like to keep it in the refrigerator, as it sets to a chewy consistency when chilled, rather like toffee.

Buckwheat honey

This honey is very dark purple, almost black in colour. The flavour is equally punchy, and suggests molasses or malt.

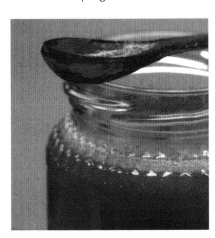

French sunflower honey

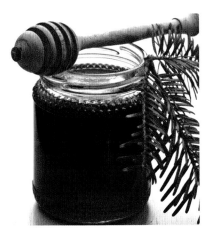

Greek pine honey

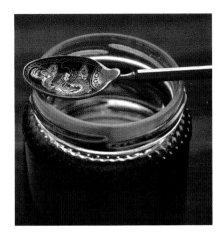

Himalayan wild flower honey

Like rapeseed honey, kiawe honey crystallizes rapidly. It must be removed from the comb at precisely the right moment. If taken too soon the water content will be too high and it may ferment; if left for too long, it will set solid. Thick and spreadable, kiawe honey has a delicate tropical flavour.

Lavender honey

Bees love lavender. Walk past a field in full flower and your ears will register the hum of thousands of happy bees, harvesting the nectar for what will become a delectable honey. Lavender honey is golden in colour, with a delicate aromatic flavour. It is sweet but relatively subtle, making it a good choice for cooking as it will not dominate.

Lehua honey

Connoisseurs of honey rave about the clean, fruity flavour of this rare Hawaiian speciality. Its source is nectar from the beautiful red flowers of the ohia tree. It is said to have a slightly salty aftertaste.

Lime/Linden/Basswood honey

All these types of honey come from trees that are members of the same family, Tilia. The common British variety, often seen in public gardens, is *Tilia europaea*. In Europe the same tree is called the linden, while an American

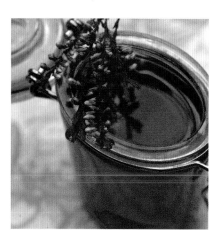

Heather honey

species is known as the basswood. Whatever the tree is called, the honey is superb. The colour – water white to pale yellow, with a greenish tinge – is not particularly exciting, but the aroma is lovely. The flavour has been likened to that of green apples with a touch of mint, and it has a definite aftertaste. Lime honey is slow to granulate.

Longan honey

Also known as dragon's eye fruit, the longan is widely cultivated in southern China, Thailand and Vietnam. Longan honey is medium to dark amber in colour, with a sweet, fruity flavour redolent of peaches.

Mesquite honey

Pale and delicately flavoured, mesquite is the most important monofloral honey produced in Mexico. The flavour has been described as citrus with a suggestion of woodsmoke. The latter is not surprising, since mesquite wood chips are widely used for barbecues.

Onion honey

One of the few honeys whose aroma is so strong that the source is undeniable. Fortunately the onion smell disappears after a few weeks, although the flavour of onion can still be detected when the pale golden honey is tasted.

Orange blossom honey

With its unmistakable citrus perfume and flavour, this is a delicious and very popular honey. The colour ranges from white to pale amber. It works well in marinades, meat glazes and as a drizzle for roasted vegetables, and is a favourite topping for ice cream, porridge, and crepes.

Rapeseed/Canola honey

The startlingly bright yellow flowers of rape (also called canola) are becoming

MANUKA HONEY

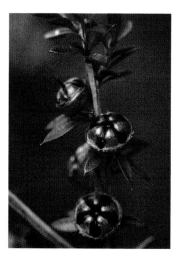

There has been a lot of media attention about this honey, most of it deserved. It is famous not for its flavour (although it does taste delicious) but for its proven antibacterial qualities. Manuka honey is produced exclusively in New Zealand, from nectar gathered from the flowers of the manuka bush (*Leptospermum scoparium* above), which grows in unpolluted areas of both North and South Island.

All honey contains hydrogen peroxide, which is a weak acid with antibacterial and anti-fungal properties. Manuka honey is no exception; it also contains a mystery phytochemical that increases its efficacy still further. For want of a better description, it has been called UMF, which simply stands for Unique Manuka Factor. When compared with a standard antiseptic, phenol (carbolic acid), active manuka honey performs extremely well. It has been claimed that it even tackles antibiotic-resistant strains of bacteria, such as MRSA.

However, it is important to note that manuka honey may only be labelled 'active' after rigorous testing. Active manuka honey sold as a foodstuff and labelled 10+ will have the same antibacterial properties as a 10 per cent phenol solution. Medical manuka honey, which should only be used externally, can be up to 20+ although 18+ is a more generally recommended strength.

Citrus-infused honey

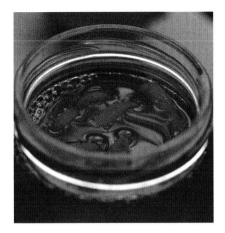

Mint-infused honey

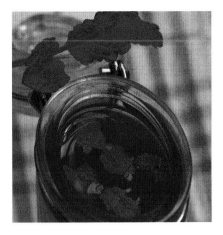

Ginger honey

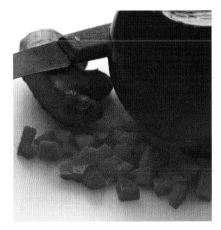

a familiar sight in many parts of the world. The set honey is white to amber and tends to be very sweet because of the high level of glucose, which makes it granulate very quickly. Rapeseed honey is used for blending and in baked goods.

Rubber honey

Rubber plantations in Sri Lanka hum with the sound of bees during the nectar flow. This occurs precisely three weeks after all leaves have dropped from the trees, making it relatively easy for beekeepers to predict when to introduce their hives. The golden or amber honey is very sweet.

Leatherwood honey

The strong, spicy, floral flavour of this unusual honey is not to everyone's taste, but it is very popular with cooks, as it is a great partner for savoury foods like chicken and lamb. The colour is a vibrant, golden yellow and the texture is creamy. Pure leatherwood honey has an enduring aftertaste that gourmets love, but those who prefer a milder flavour can opt for a blended version.

Rosemary honey

This is a very pale honey with a subtle, herby aroma. It comes from the mountains of Catalonia in eastern Spain and the lavender fields of Provence.

Sunflower honey

A warm, yellow colour, sunflower honey sets soon after being removed from the comb. The set honey is thick and creamy. It is widely produced and is especially popular in France and Italy. The flavour is not too sweet, with a light lemon tang.

Thyme honey

The most famous thyme honey is Hymettus, named after a mountain in ancient Greece whose thyme bushes produced honey of such quality that it was called the food of the gods. Thyme honey has a robust herbal flavour. It is golden in colour, with a reddish tinge.

Tupelo honey

The tupelo or pepperidge tree is native to eastern North America and also grows in southern Asia. In northern Florida hives are kept on platforms along the river swamps. Tupelo honey is golden in colour, with a greenish cast. It is much sought-after because of its lovely floral perfume and complex, somewhat fruity flavour and aftertaste. The honey has such a high ratio of fructose to glucose that it is very slow to crystallize.

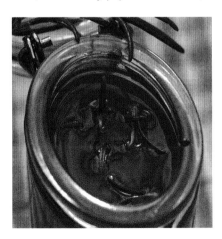

Rosemary honey

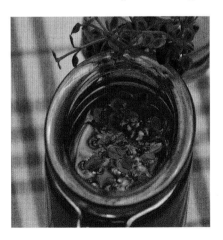

Thyme honey

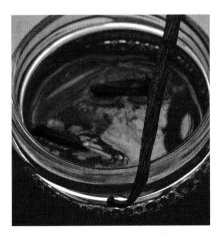

Vanilla honey

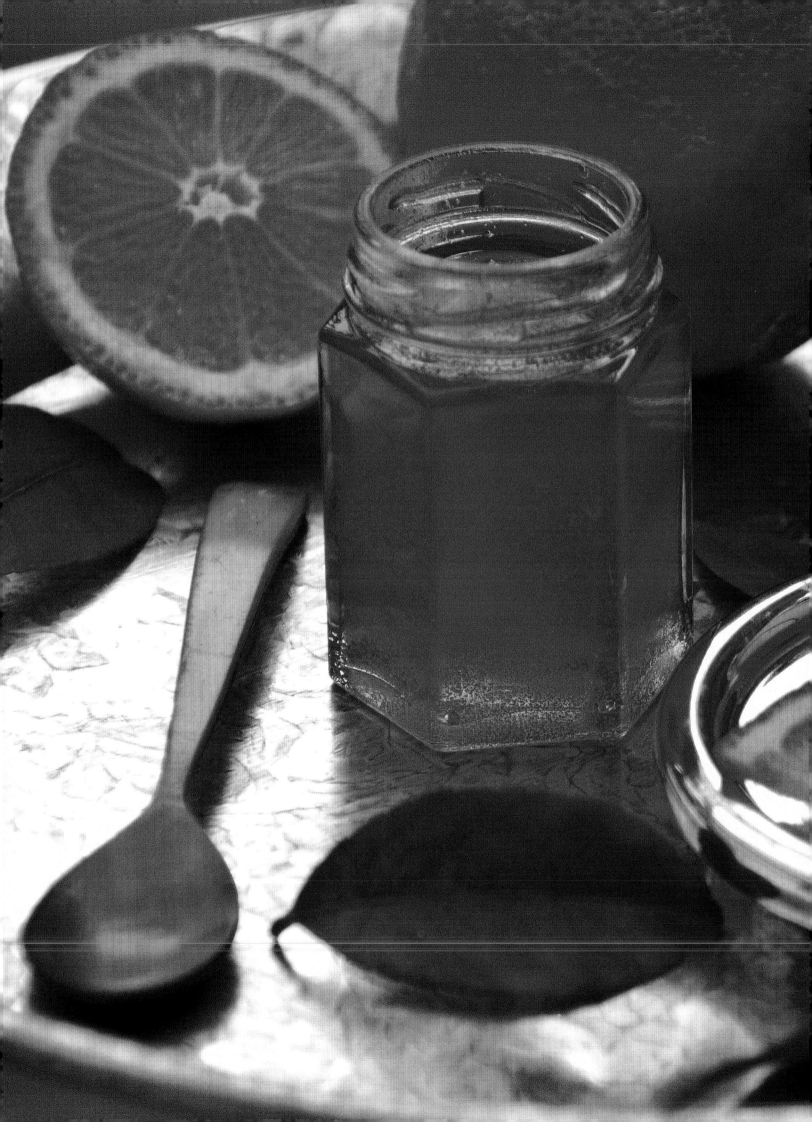

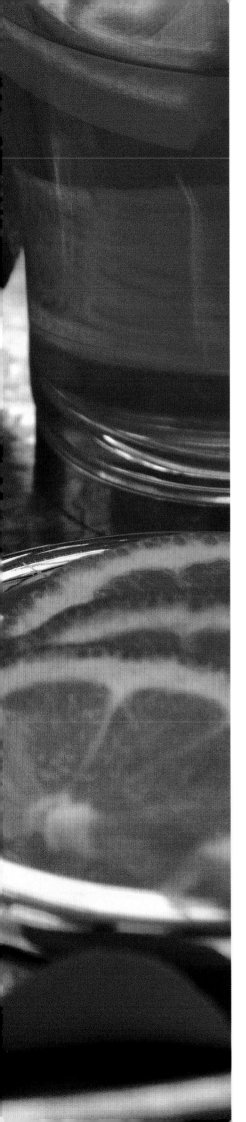

HONEY FOR HEALTH AND HEALING

There is nothing new about the link between honey and health. People the world over have long recognized honey's therapeutic qualities. Honey is just a concentrated solution of sugars in water, but it also contains amino acids, proteins, minerals and vitamins. Nutritionally, these are insignificant, but they appear to play a part in helping some medical conditions. There is increasing evidence of honey's efficacy in treating wounds and burns, and manuka honey is an effective antibacterial agent.

Left: Honey and lemon is a tried and tested remedy for sore throats owing to the antiseptic and antibacterial properties of honey.

AN ANCIENT AND MODERN REMEDY

Ancient Sumerians, Greeks, Egyptians and Phoenicians all used honey for healing. It played, and still plays, an important role in both Ayurvedic and traditional Islamic medicine.

None of the current research into the benefits of honey would unduly surprise the ancient Egyptians, for whom honey was an everyday remedy. Transcripts of some of the earliest records, papyruses dating back four thousand years or more, list honey as a prime ingredient in prescriptions for hundreds of conditions. For stomach pain, constipation and urinary retention, patients were advised to take honey orally, while pastes and ointments were made up for the treatment of ulcers, sores and wounds. Practitioners in both Sumeria and Egypt routinely used salves made from honey to promote healing after ear-piercing and circumcision.

Honey was also used to treat burns. One practice, used by the ancient Egyptians and being revived today, was to impregnate strips of linen with honey and place them over the affected area. The honey promoted healing and prevented sepsis from setting in.

Honey is an anti-inflammatory, and Egyptians used it for the treatment of strains and stiff joints. Their physicians prescribed a honey salve for eye infections and also recommended honey for the treatment of ulcers. Honey was even prescribed as a cure for baldness, although its efficacy in this area has not been proven.

Honey and the ancients

The ancient Greeks liked to eat honey, but they used it medicinally as well. Hippocrates prescribed honey for ulcers and sores. Aristotle claimed that those who regularly ate honey lived longer, a belief with which the philosopher Democritus, concurred. We are told that he lived for over a hundred years and attributed his great age in an era where many died young to a daily massage with olive oil and a regular diet of honey. Al-Razi, the famous Persian philosopher and physician, commended honey and vinegar for the treatment of various disorders, including gum disease and skin irritation. His belief in the efficacy of honey was not unusual in the Muslim world. The Qur'an, or Koran, the Islamic holy book, devotes an entire chapter to bees and honey, describing the latter as "a drink diverse of hues, where is healing for mankind."

Chinese medicine

Honey is also highlighted in Chinese traditional medicine. Li Shizhen, who recorded the formulations of over a thousand herbal medicines during the Ming Dynasty, suggested that medicinal herbs should be roasted with honey to improve their effectiveness. For a wheezy cough, the bulbs of a certain type of lily were ground to a powder with coltsfood flowers, then bound with honey.

The advent of antibiotics

Honey continued to be used regularly until the early 20th century, when more sophisticated medical treatments and the discovery of antibiotics caused it to fall from favour. In 1910 it was still being recommended for a variety of minor medical conditions.

The discovery of penicillin and the sulfonamide drugs diverted attention from honey for decades, but antibiotic-resistant drugs like MRSA and Group A streptococcus has put it back in the limelight. It has been claimed that manuka honey is a safe long-term treatment option until the infection is cleared.

Above: This papyrus, c.1539–1292BCE, is 18th-dynasty New Kingdom Egyptian. It describes a medicinal recipe containing honey as "another perfect remedy."

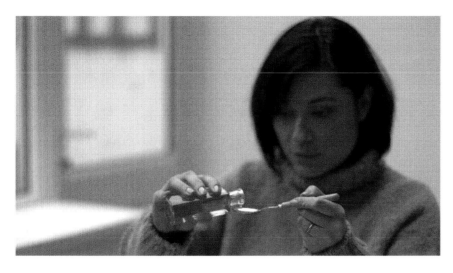

Above: When mixed with lemon juice or vinegar, honey is a tried-and-tested remedy for irritating conditions such as coughs, colds and sore throats.

How honey heals

Honey promotes healing in a variety of ways. The high sugar and low moisture levels create an osmotic effect, drawing liquid out of anything that comes into contact with it. If this is a bacterium, it is desiccated and dies. The same hygroscopic effect (ability to absorb and hold moisture) means that excess fluids are drawn from the wound site, which helps to reduce oedema (build up of fluid in tissues) and inflammation. Added to this, honey is acidic, which creates an inhospitable environment for bacteria. Finally, honey is a source of hydrogen peroxide, which is a well-known antiseptic. Dilute the honey (by moisture from a wound, for instance) and the enzyme kicks in again, giving the antibacterial activity in the honey a massive boost. The honey carries on working efficiently, even though the hydrogen peroxide is much less concentrated than a standard 3 per cent antiseptic solution. The honey is gentler and will not harm tissues.

Honey in healing

Ulcers, bedsores, abscesses, boils, burns and post-operative infections have all been treated successfully with honey and it has been used for wounds that refuse to heal, even after a year. Doctors working at Bonn University Children's Hospital reported good results after using medical honey to treat chronic wounds in children with cancer. A double-blind controlled trial among gold miners in South Africa concluded that honey was safe and as effective as a commercial healing gel in treating wounds and abrasions.

Active manuka honey is especially successful in fighting bacteria, owing to an ingredient called UMF (unique manuka factor). Manuka honey for medical purposes is packaged in tubes in New Zealand, where the manuka bush grows. It is used in burn and wound dressings, which are effective and popular with patients, since they do not stick to the wound and also have a deodorizing quality. Manuka dressings have been in use in British and Australian hospitals for some time, and have now become accepted in Canada and the United States.

Honey and hay fever

Symptoms of hay fever vary: some people have streaming eyes, runny noses and tight chests. In recent years there has been a lot of discussion about whether honey can help hay fever sufferers. The theory is if a locally produced unfiltered honey with small amounts of pollen is eaten regularly, immunity will build up to pollen from plants that grow in that area. Honeycomb is said to be even more effective than liquid honey. Anecdotal evidence also suggests that taking a teaspoon of local honey every day before the start of the hay fever season can be successful. Nettle tea, sweetened with honey, is also recommended for hay fever sufferers.

THERAPEUTIC BEE STINGS

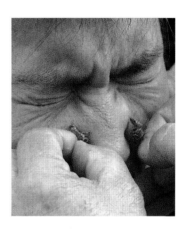

The idea of being deliberately stung by bees may seem strange, but there are claims that bee venom can help to alleviate the symptoms of arthritis and multiple sclerosis. The theory is that the localised inflammation caused by the stings triggers an anti-inflammatory response and the release of a natural painkiller, cortisol. Patients have regular sessions, some being stung up to forty times on each occasion. There is anecdotal evidence that some sufferers have improved after they were given bee venom, however, scientific proof is scanty and MS organizations counsel individuals to check with their doctor or neurologist before considering this type of treatment. One concern is the risk of anaphylactic shock, a life-threatening allergic reaction.

HONEY REMEDIES FOR RESPIRATORY CONDITIONS

Honey is acknowledged by modern science to have antibacterial properties and deters the growth of some bacteria. It is also soothing for sore throats and coughs.

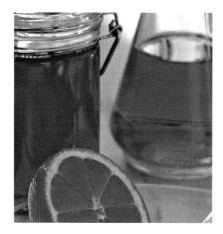

Coughs and colds

Honey is universally used for relief from bronchial ailments such as coughs and colds and has been used by Greeks, Italians and Hungarians for centuries. Together with the antibacterial properties of vinegar, it provides a powerful antidote. Take one teaspoon as needed to help quieten a cough.

INGREDIENTS

5ml/1 tsp lemon juice

5ml/1 tsp honey

5ml/1 tsp vinegar

1 Mix lemon, honey and vinegar.

2 Take one teaspoon every 2–3 hours or when needed.

MAKING REMEDIES

• When preparing remedies, use glass or stainless steel bowls and utensils – not wood or plastic.

• If possible use dried herbs.

• Refrigerate the mixture if no preservatives are used.

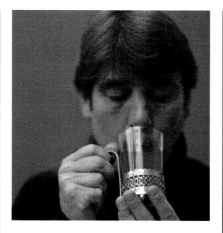

Sore throats

A mugful of this healing winter remedy, taken twice a day, will relieve and prevent sore throats, or sip a teaspoon slowly at night before going to bed.

INGREDIENTS

1.5ml/$\frac{1}{4}$ tsp cayenne pepper

2.5ml/$\frac{1}{2}$ tsp ground ginger

15ml/1 tbsp honey

1 Mix together all the ingredients in a cup or mug.

2 Fill up with hot water.

3 Take one sip at a time.

LARYNGITIS

To make a drink to soothe a sore throat: Peel a 2.5-cm/1-in piece of fresh root ginger. Slice it very thinly and discard the woody centre of the ginger. Place 6–8 ginger shavings in a cup and add boiling water to fill the cup. Stir in 15ml/1 tbsp honey. Leave to stand until lukewarm before drinking, or if you prefer, chill and then drink cold.

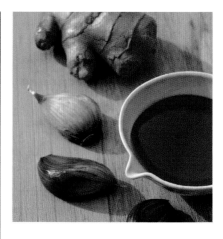

Respiratory problems

Honey is believed to help relieve hay fever, and it may help the immune system achieve a better resistance to airborne allergies.

INGREDIENTS

5ml/1 tsp honey

2.5ml/$\frac{1}{2}$ tsp ground ginger

2.5ml/$\frac{1}{2}$ tsp crushed garlic

1 In a small bowl, mix together the honey, ginger and garlic.

2 Take with a teaspoon or dilute in a cup of water.

HAY FEVER

Pollen has been effectively used throughout the ages to relieve asthma sufferers. The treatment consisted of giving small amounts of the allergen that stimulated the asthmatic's immune system to produce antibodies, to fight the allergic reaction. Pollen is also useful for reducing the effects of hay fever; it must be taken six weeks or more before and during the length of the season.

HONEY REMEDIES FOR INTERRUPTED SLEEP

Whether sleep is disrupted by insomnia or by bedwetting, regular use of a spoonful of honey at bedtime may help remedy the condition.

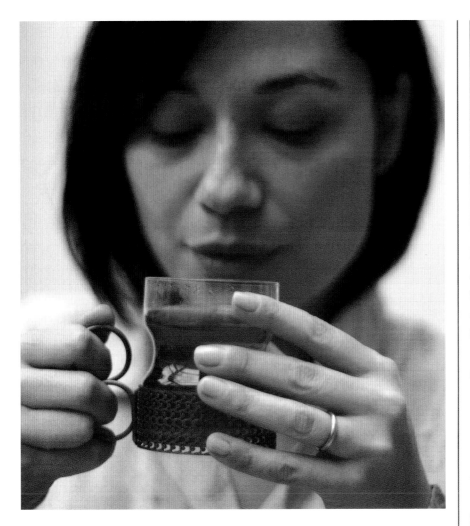

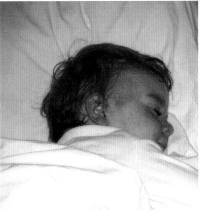

Bedwetting

A tablespoon of honey given at bedtime is an old remedy used to reduce and put a stop to bedwetting. No liquids for three hours before going to bed will also help.

INGREDIENTS

15ml/1 tbsp honey

1 Swallow the honey.

2 Brush teeth before going to bed.

Insomnia

The route to a good night's sleep is to drink a tranquillizing beverage just before bedtime.

Mild or transient insomnia can be helped with natural remedies, however if the sleeplessness is chronic it could be caused by an underlying problem that needs medical attention, such as depression or heart disease.

Camomile has a component called chrysin that can promote sleep and can be used in conjunction with honey to relieve insomnia.

INGREDIENTS

5ml/1 tsp honey
a handful of fresh or dried mint leaves
250ml/8fl oz/1 cup camomile tea

1 Add the honey and the mint leaves to the camomile tea.

2 Leave to soak for a while to extract the mint flavour.

3 Strain the tea into a jug and discard the leaves. Sip a cup of the tea just before going to bed each evening.

SEDATIVE

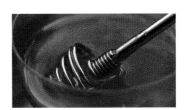

Honey has a mild sedative effect and it holds fluid in a child's body while he or she sleeps. Honey should never be given to infants under the age of one because it contains bacteria that can be dangerous to infants (but harmless to adults and older children).

HONEY REMEDIES FOR EXPECTANT MOTHERS

Two common complaints during pregnancy are anaemia and morning sickness. For relief try the simple remedies here, but if severe, always consult your doctor for advice.

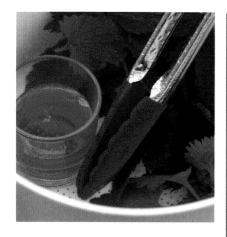

Anaemia

Women who are vegetarian are often affected by anaemia because they are unable to increase their iron intake by eating meat products. However, they can introduce more iron into their diet by eating nettles. Pick only young nettles that grow away from roads. Always wear rubber gloves to handle the nettles.

INGREDIENTS

10ml/2 tsp honey

200g/8oz/4 cups young nettle tops

1 Steam the nettle tops for a few minutes until they are limp.

2 Drain the nettle tops and transfer them to a serving plate, then drizzle with the honey.

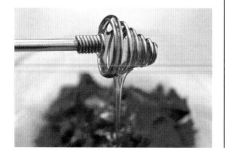

Morning sickness

This common condition affects 60 to 80 per cent of all women during their first trimester. A new research study has shown that a mixture of ginger and honey is a safe and effective way to treat morning sickness. If the sickness is severe, omit the bran and add the honey and ginger to spring water and take as a drink.

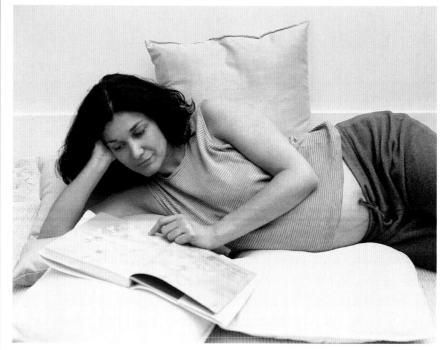

INGREDIENTS

15ml/1 tbsp honey

5ml/1 tsp root ginger, peeled
  and sliced

bran (or water if the sickness is severe)

1 Mix the honey and ginger in a bowl.

2 Add the bran and eat as a cereal.

HEARTBURN

Many pregnant women suffer from heartburn. For relief, mix 5ml/1 tsp honey with a glass of milk to neutralize excess acid.

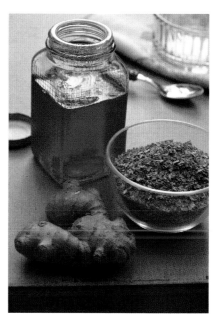

HONEY REMEDIES FOR DIGESTIVE PROBLEMS

Honey is easily digested and has long been recognized as a remedy for stomach or intestinal problems. If someone is feeling off-colour, it gives a quick lift and improves the appetite.

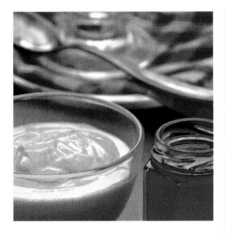

Diarrhoea

This remedy for diarrhoea or vomiting, or both, works fast. If you only feel able to take liquids, just drink a glass of barley water with a teaspoon of honey added. As the ingredients are easily available, it provides quick relief for stomach upsets.

INGREDIENTS

225g/8oz/1 cup natural (plain) yogurt
15ml/1 tbsp honey

1 Stir the yogurt and honey together.

2 Eat the remedy when required.

HANGOVERS

Dr Martensen-Larsen, a leading expert on alcoholism, believes that honey aids the recovery from hangovers by blocking the route of alcohol to the brain, raising blood sugar levels and stimulating the elimination of waste and toxins. Mix 250ml/8fl oz/1 cup dandelion or nettle tea with 10ml/2 tsp honey. Stir and drink.

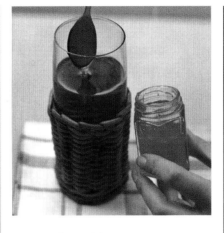

Stomach problems

Often the cause of stomach upsets is the *heliocobacter pylori* bacteria. Honey is known to inhibit the growth of this strain, so much so that it is sometimes advised for the relief of ulcers. It is administered each evening before bedtime. Nettle, used in this remedy because it is a natural diuretic, also stimulates the digestive system to combat any problems.

INGREDIENTS

250ml/8fl oz/1 cup nettle tea
10ml/2 tsp honey

1 Make a cup of nettle tea in a heatproof glass or mug.

2 Stir in the honey to sweeten.

STOMACH ACHE

Mix 15ml/1 tbsp honey with 15ml/1 tbsp lemon or 10ml/ 2 tsp cider vinegar. Add hot water and stir well before drinking. This drink can relieve stomach ache and indigestion.

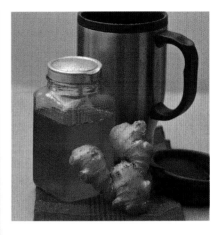

Travel sickness

Ginger has an anti-emetic property owing to its aromatic oil, which also gives ginger its flavour. A flask of ginger tea infused with honey, or water flavoured with ginger, is useful for passengers prone to travel sickness.

INGREDIENTS

15ml/1 tbsp honey
15ml/1 tbsp ground ginger or 2.5cm/1in fresh root ginger, peeled and sliced
1 litre/1¾ pints/4 cups ginger tea or hot water

1 Mix the honey and ginger together.

2 Add to ginger tea or hot water and decant to a flask. If using fresh ginger, remove and discard.

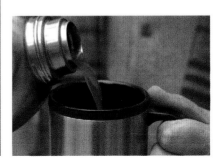

HONEY REMEDIES FOR STRESSFUL CONDITIONS

Honey is believed to be a stabilizer, calming highs and helping through low points. Because it is made of simple sugars, honey is easily digested and quickly increases energy levels.

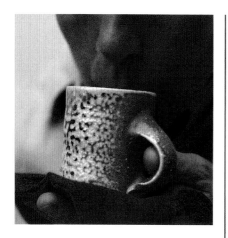

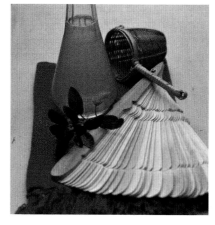

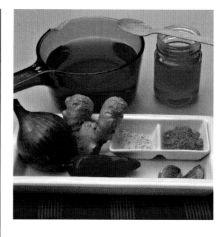

Nerves

A tablespoon of ginseng elixir every day before breakfast or a cup of ginseng and honey in water will relax the nerves and help in the recovery of any damage to the nervous system, in preparation for the pressures of the day ahead.

INGREDIENTS

5ml/1 tsp powdered ginseng

5ml/1 tsp honey

250ml/8fl oz/1 cup hot water

1 Mix the ginseng and honey together, then add the hot water.

2 Allow to stand for 1 minute before drinking.

LISTLESSNESS

Reach for the honey instead of a chocolate bar if you are running out of steam. The fructose and glucose in honey are easily digested and will give a rapid boost. Try a spoonful of honey before a gym workout. After an energetic session, refuel with a banana and honey sandwich.

Hot flushes

These can be an embarrassing symptom of the menopause, lasting months and sometimes years. The face flushes in colour followed by drenching sweat and an aftermath of cold and clamminess. It can be relieved by wearing light clothes and keeping a flow of air through the house or office. Regular drinks of this mix can relieve symptoms, and the sage content can help with excess sweating and the rebalancing of hormones.

INGREDIENTS

15ml/1 tbsp honey

10ml/2 tsp lemon juice

10ml/2 tsp dried sage

5ml/1 tsp dried angelica

1 litre/1¾ pints/4 cups water

1 Put the honey, lemon juice, sage and angelica in a pan with the water. Bring to the boil and simmer over a low heat for 5–10 minutes. Leave to cool.

2 Strain and pour the mixture into a bottle. Refrigerate until required then drink regularly to relieve the symptoms.

Low energy

This tonic will lift the spirits and energy levels according to traditional Chinese medicine. The following infusion, to be taken as needed, will stimulate the circulatory system, increase the efficiency of the body's blood and lymph flow and increase the feeling of wellbeing.

INGREDIENTS

1 litre/1¾ pints/4 cups cider vinegar or herbal tea of choice

15ml/1 tbsp finely chopped onion

2 cloves garlic, finely chopped

15ml/1 tbsp fresh ginger, peeled and sliced

1 jalepeño pepper, seeded and chopped

5ml/1 tsp grated horseradish

15ml/1 tbsp honey

1 Mix the cider vinegar, the chopped onion, garlic, ginger, jalapeño pepper, horseradish and honey in a saucepan.

2 Bring to the boil and simmer for about 10 minutes.

3 Cool, strain and store in the refrigerator.

Migraine and headaches

Caused by a tightening of the soft tissue covering the skull, migraines and headaches are often triggered by stress and hormonal changes, which can be aggravated by foods such as chocolate and red wine. An infusion of calming herbs and tea, together with nutritious honey to sweeten it, can help calm this tension. To prevent an attack of migraine, take 10ml/2 tsp honey at mealtimes.

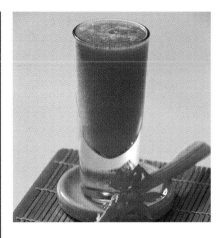

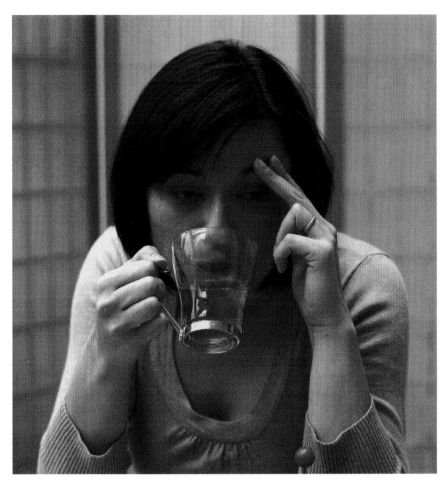

INGREDIENTS

10ml/2 tsp dried melissa

10ml/2 tsp dried peppermint

10ml/2 tsp dried yarrow

5ml/1 tsp dried camomile

10ml/2 tsp honey

475ml/16floz/2 cups green tea

1 Mix the dried melissa, peppermint, yarrow, camomile and honey into the green tea. Leave to soak for 5–10 minutes.

2 Strain, transfer the remedy to a glass and take a small cup every 2 hours.

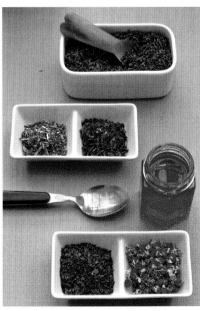

Tension

The potassium in honey is thought to be a relaxant, and celery contains active compounds called pthalides, which aid the relaxation of the muscles of the arteries that regulate blood pressure. At the same time the amount of stress hormones are lowered so that tension is reduced. A tablespoon of this relaxant at mealtimes can have a very beneficial effect in promoting relaxation and reducing nervous tension.

INGREDIENTS

4 celery sticks

15ml/1 tbsp honey

15ml/1 tbsp water

1 Chop the celery into small pieces, then liquidize with the honey and water until well blended. Add a little more water, if necessary, to make a smooth drink.

2 Pour some relaxant into a glass and refrigerate the remainder until required.

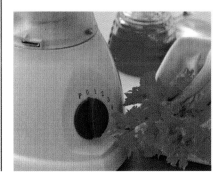

HONEY REMEDIES FOR SKIN CONDITIONS

Honey is known for is anti-microbial activity and in some cases it appears to work quicker than conventional treatments, particularly for burns and bedsores.

Bedsores

Rhubarb has been used medicinally since 3000BCE, and with honey it helps to heal bedsores when a paste is applied to the affected area. Cook a stick of rhubarb until soft and strain the juice.

INGREDIENTS

15ml/1 tbsp honey

15ml/1 tbsp rhubarb juice

clean lint

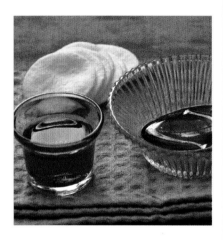

1 In a small bowl, mix the honey and rhubarb juice together.

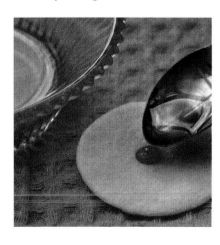

2 Spread the paste on a piece of clean lint and apply to the sore.

Burns

Research shows that burns treated with honey-soaked gauze heal twice as quickly as those employing orthodox methods, and scarring was reduced. Honey inhibits fungi and bacteria.

INGREDIENTS

15ml/1 tbsp honey or propolis

sterilized gauze

tape

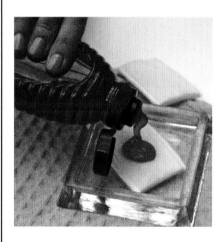

1 Spread honey or propolis on a piece of sterilized gauze.

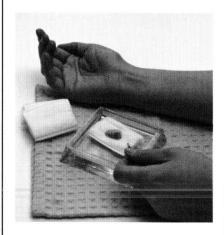

2 Apply the gauze to the burn, then secure with tape.

Grazes and sores

This simple remedy uses a dab of honey, which is sealed with petroleum or royal jelly. The honey kills the bacteria and speeds healing of the graze or sore, while the jelly excludes air and helps to keep the skin sterile.

INGREDIENTS

5ml/1 tsp honey

a little petroleum jelly or royal jelly

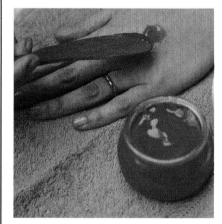

1 Cover the graze or sore with a small dab of honey.

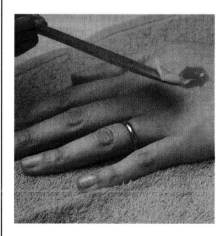

2 Seal with petroleum or royal jelly and leave overnight.

Sunburn

As well as being good at treating burns, honey also helps to heal sunburn. Used straight from the refrigerator, this cream makes a very soothing after-sun treatment, applied to affected areas. Any redness will be calmed by the anti-inflammatory properties of the aloe vera, which also acts as an analgesic.

INGREDIENTS

20ml/4 tsp beeswax granules

60ml/4 tbsp honey

10ml/2 tsp aloe vera or wheat germ oil

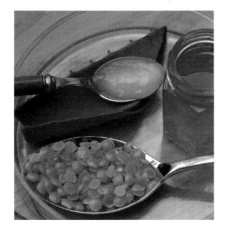

1 Put the beeswax granules with the honey and aloe vera gel or oil in a warmed bowl.

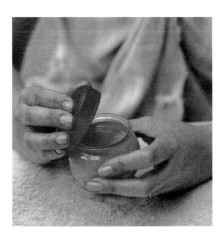

2 Stir well to mix and, if necessary, warm again in a bain marie to melt the beeswax. Transfer the mixture to a wide-necked jar and gently smooth on to skin to soothe sunburn.

Cuts

Because honey is rich in sugar, vitamins, minerals and enzymes including inhibine, which helps to prevent infection, it can be used as an antibiotic ointment for wounds. A research trial published in the British Journal of Plastic Surgery proved that as germs did not survive in honey, it proved to be a faster wound healer than a specifically trialled hospital product.

INGREDIENTS

5ml/1 tsp honey or propolis

cotton wool balls, lint and bandage

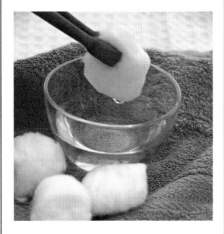

1 Soak cotton wool balls in water, then use them to clean the wound. Hold them in tongs to keep sterile.

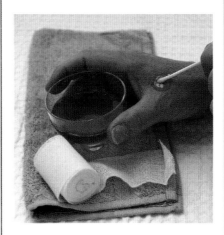

2 Use a cotton bud to apply honey or propolis to the wound. Cover the area with a sterile wrap or sterilized lint followed by a bandage. Check the next day and replace if necessary.

Dry skin

As well as having antibacterial and antibiotic properties, honey has a healing and moisturizing effect on dry skin, stimulating regrowth and renewal. This simple exfoliating remedy can be made using ingredients from the kitchen storecupboard.

INGREDIENTS

30ml/2 tbsp honey

30ml/2 tbsp olive oil

30ml/2 tbsp natural (plain) yogurt

45ml/3 tbsp pinhead oatmeal

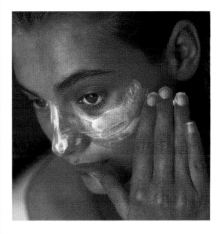

1 Mix all the ingredients together to make a paste and apply gently to the face, avoiding the eye area.

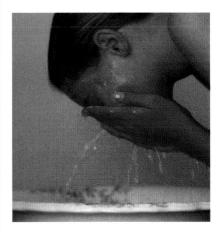

2 Leave the paste on for 5 minutes, then wash off with warm water. Finish by splashing the face with cool water to refresh the skin and boost the circulation to the face.

HONEY REMEDIES FOR WEIGHT LOSS AND ENERGY

Taking honey is reputed to induce a feeling of fullness so is a good food to help slimming. Honey also gives a boost to energy and is thought to support the immune system.

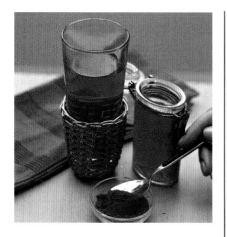

Slimming

Honey mixed with cinnamon is claimed to help in weight loss. Unlike sugar, honey contains vitamins and minerals, which are believed to help in fat and cholesterol metabolism. Using honey instead of sugar can reduce calories.

INGREDIENTS

15ml/1 tbsp honey

2.5ml/½ tsp ground cinnamon

1 Mix the ingredients in a cup.

2 Add boiling water and stir. Cool a little before drinking.

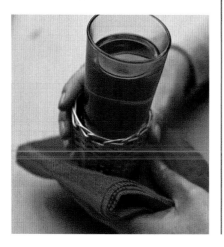

Energy boost and immune support

Fruit sugars in honey are easily digested to provide a natural energy boost for the body. Honey-based drinks are an alternative to those that enhance athletic performance, at the same time replacing body minerals lost through perspiration.

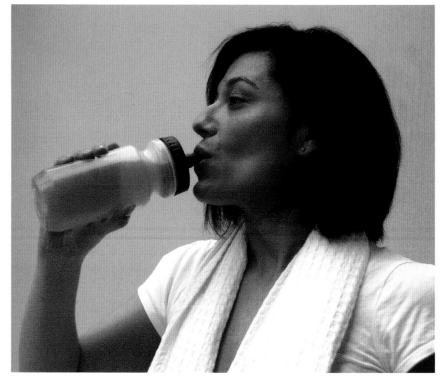

INGREDIENTS

45ml/3 tbsp honey

5ml/1 tsp each salt and cider vinegar

1 Mix the ingredients together.

2 Add to a flask with water. Shake well.

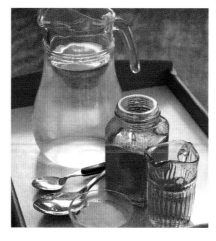

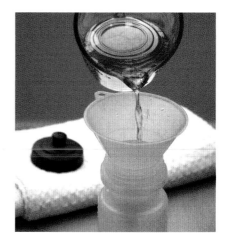

HONEY REMEDIES FOR AILMENTS IN OLDER LIFE

As people age, ailments and health problems tend to appear. Remedies using honey and beeswax that have been tried and tested over decades can offer relief in a natural way.

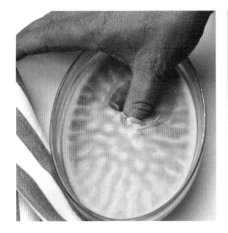

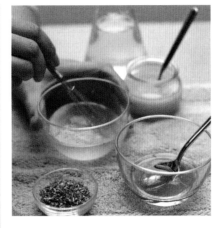

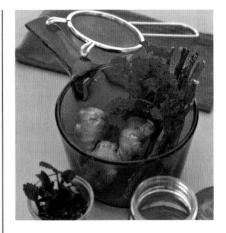

Arthritis

There have been many documented cases of arthritis sufferers finding relief from wax treatments to affected parts. The hot wax eases stiffness caused by inflammation of the joints.

INGREDIENTS
2.25kg/5lb beeswax
475ml/16fl oz/2 cups mineral oil

1 Heat the oven to 100°C/200°/Gas ¼. Place the beeswax and mineral oil in an ovenproof dish and heat in the oven until the wax has melted. Stir occasionally to blend the wax and oil.

2 Carefully remove from the oven and allow to cool until the mixture is still warm but not uncomfortably hot. Dip the part of the body to be treated into the wax mixture then withdraw when it is coated in wax. If you are treating the hand, keep the fingers apart.

3 Repeat until there is a thick coating, then leave in the wax until the mixture cools. Remove and peel off the wax.

Hair restorer

Once a day, massaging the scalp rigorously with the fingertips in a shampooing action will activate the sebaceous glands, stimulate the hair follicles and generally improve the circulation of blood to the affected area. This preparation, used weekly, will nourish the hair with vitamins and minerals that may be lacking in the diet. You should start to see a marked improvement after a few weeks and the hair should look glowing and healthy.

INGREDIENTS
5ml/1 tsp honey
2.5ml/½ tsp olive oil
5ml/1 tsp dried sage
90ml/6 tbsp mineral water

1 Add the honey, olive oil and sage to the mineral water and mix well.

2 Massage the mixture into the scalp for a few minutes.

3 Leave the preparation on the head for about 30 minutes, then wash off.

Gall stones

Caused by a build-up of calcifications in the gall bladder, gall stones can be small and easy to pass, or may be painful and require medical attention. An old country remedy to reduce the likelihood of stones increasing in size is to drink a measure of this herbal mix daily.

INGREDIENTS
1 litre/1¾ pints/4 cups water
25ml/1½ tbsp honey
15ml/1 tbsp ground ginger
25ml/1½ tbsp lemon balm
25ml/1½ tbsp freshly chopped parsley
15g/½ oz liquorice root

1 Boil the water in a pan and add the honey, ginger, lemon balm, parsley and liquorice root.

2 Bring to the boil, then simmer until the volume is reduced by half.

3 Leave to cool, then strain into a bottle and store in the refrigerator.

4 Drink a glass of the mixture every day.

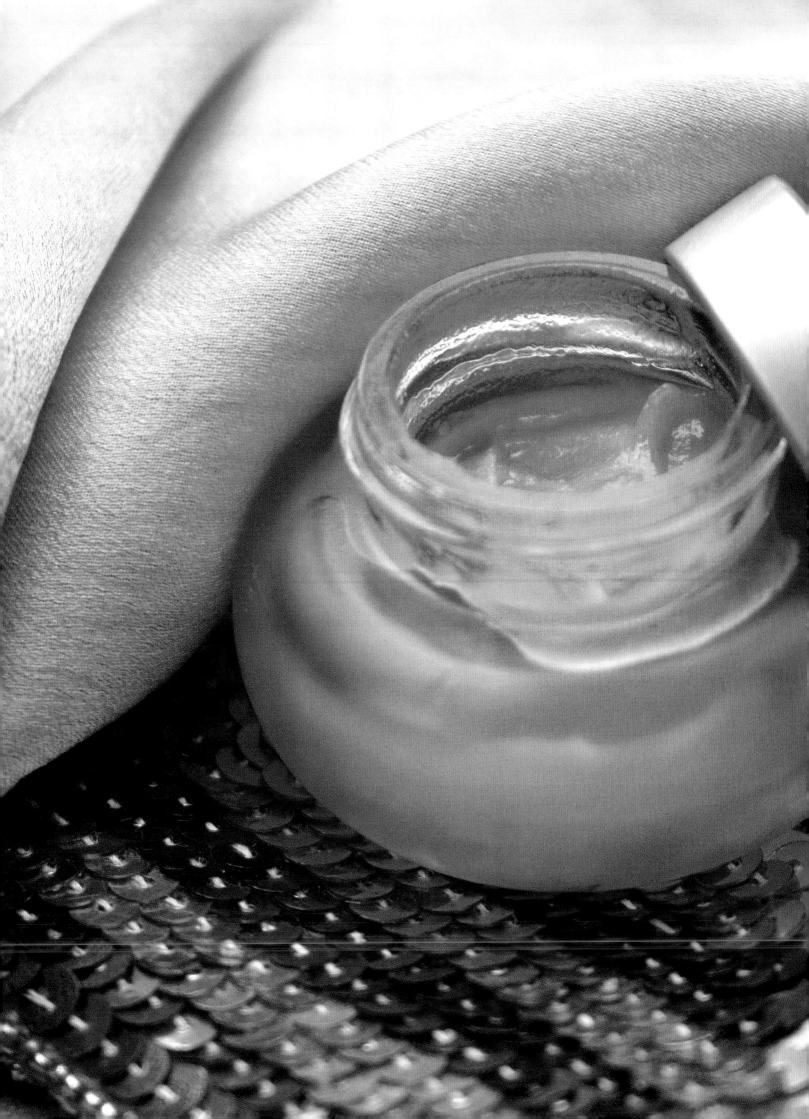

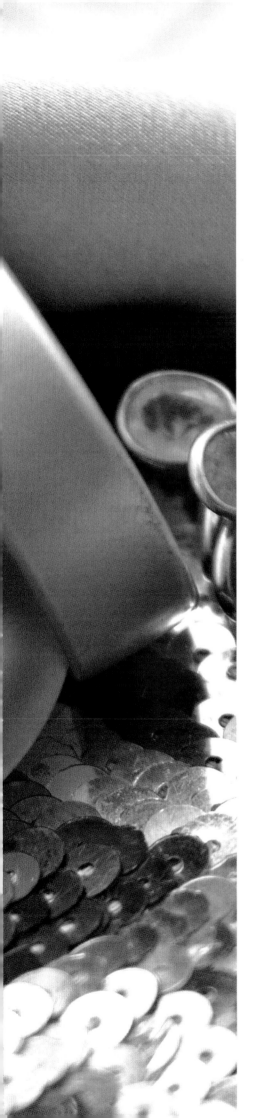

NATURAL BEAUTY WITH HONEY AND BEESWAX

Honey has been used as a beauty preparation since the days of the ancient Romans – and for a lot longer than that. In the days of the pharaohs, honey was used in face washes, hair rinses and potions. To promote soft skin and a radiant complexion, a honey mask was applied by Egyptian ladies, and beeswax was used in wrinkle creams and pomades. The qualities of honey and beeswax are still recognized and they are just as relevant today in beauty products.

Left: Beeswax is used to set this solid perfume, which can be divided into small containers and carried in a handbag.

HONEY FOR SCENTS AND BATHING

Using honey in a bath balm will leave the skin smooth and soothed, combating any dryness. Beeswax is the base for the solid perfume, which is easy to carry around without spilling.

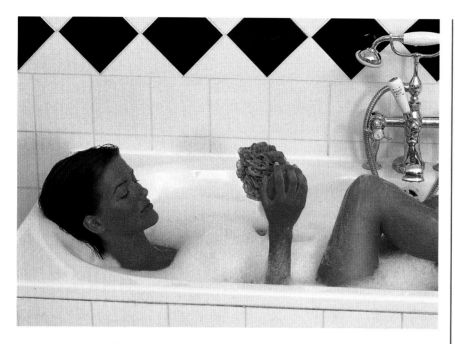

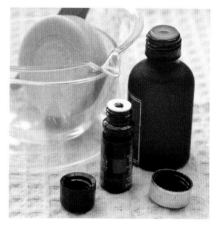

Honey and vanilla bath oil

If you prefer bubbles in your bath you can replace 100ml/3½fl oz/½ cup of oil with liquid soap or 115g/4oz of hand-made soap. Have a different oil each day of the week by replacing the vanilla and lemon with essential oils. Try lavender for relaxation, patchouli for a heavily scented, pampering bath or a mix to suit.

INGREDIENTS

350ml/12fl oz/1½ cups jojoba or sweet
  almond oil
120ml/4fl oz/½ cup honey
15ml/1 tbsp vanilla extract
15ml/1 tbsp lemon juice

1 Pour all the oil into a suitable bowl and slowly add the other ingredients, stirring gently. You may wish to slightly warm the honey beforehand to speed up the blending process.

2 Put the mixture into a coloured bottle with a tight-fitting lid to stop deterioration from exposure to light. Remember to shake the bottle gently before using.

3 Store the oil in a cool, dark place.

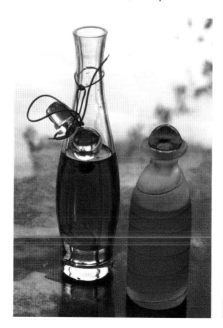

Solid perfume

Add your favourite essential oil or scent to this perfume. You may wish to make a large quantity and decant into several small containers or to make small quantities with different perfumes, so the recipe is given in parts. For example a small 6g pot would consist of 3g oil, 2g wax and 1g essential oil or scent.

INGREDIENTS

3 parts jojoba or sweet almond oil
2 parts beeswax, preferably white
1 part essential oil or scent

1 In a bain marie, heat the jojoba or almond oil, beeswax and oils or scent.

2 Stir with a wooden spoon and pour into a jar or container.

SCENTED OILS

Ring the changes with different essential oils. The use of grapefruit would uplift the spirits, whereas ylang ylang and bergamot would create a very sensual smell.

Bath bombs

These are very easy to make, are fun and will leave the bathroom filled with a wonderful aroma. Simply drop them in the tub and the ingredients will explode, releasing all their scent and petals. Children suddenly find bathing a time to look forward to and can have fun making their own bombs. Wrapped in coloured cellophane, foil or brown paper and tied with ribbon or raffia, they make inexpensive, attractive gifts.

INGREDIENTS

225g/8oz/1 cup bicarbonate of soda
  (baking soda)
90g/3½oz/½ cup citric acid
15ml/1 tbsp honey
few drops vanilla extract or essential oil
150ml/¼ pint/⅔ cup witch hazel, decanted
  into a spray bottle
15ml/1 tbsp dried herbs, petals, or food
  colouring (optional)

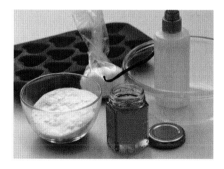

1 Mix the bicarbonate of soda and citric acid in a bowl until blended.

2 Add the honey and vanilla or essential oil, to perfume the mixture.

3 Add any optional ingredients, such as the herbs or petals and a chosen food colouring. Work quickly to avoid the bomb exploding prematurely. Using the witch hazel spray, spritz the mixture until wet and stir with your hand until it reaches a dough-like consistency.

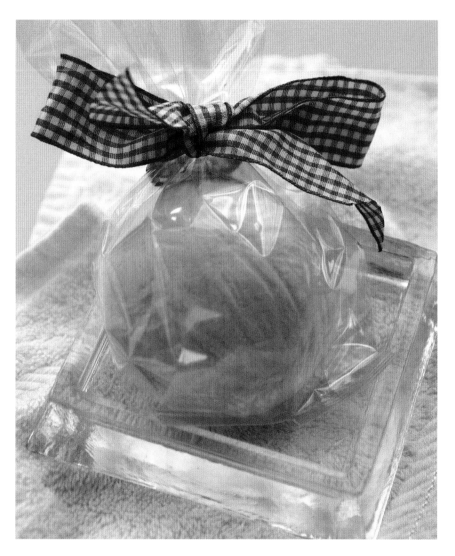

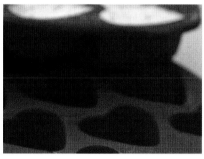

4 If the mixture starts to fizz, add a little more of the bicarbonate of soda, which will take up the extra witch hazel. Press the mixture into a mould such as an ice-cube tray, or roll into balls and place on a tray or board. Leave overnight to dry out thoroughly.

5 For a special gift, make a large bomb, wrap it in cellophane and tie a pretty ribbon around it.

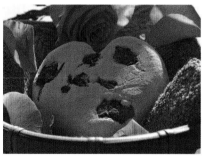

TIP

The tighter you pack the mixture into the moulds, the harder and longer lasting the bomb will turn out. As with baking recipes, after you have made the bombs a few time, you will be better able to judge the approximate quantities of the dry ingredient and the witch hazel. This will allow you to get the best consistency for your bombs.

HONEY FOR HAIRCARE

With honey and a few simple ingredients, you can make natural shampoos and conditioner for most hair types that will leave your hair clean and shining.

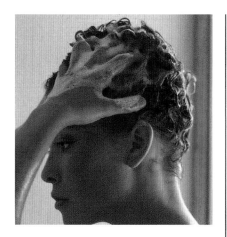

Normal shampoo

Many hair products today base their ingredients on natural products. One of the first of these was the famous egg shampoo based on a very old recipe that is easy to follow at home. With the addition of honey, this rich shampoo leaves the hair healthy and shiny.

INGREDIENTS

1 large egg
5ml/1 tsp honey
45ml/3 tbsp soap flakes

1 Separate the yolk and white of the egg. Whisk the egg white until frothy.

2 Blend in the yolk and honey and add the soap flakes. Wet the hair with warm water – do not use hot water as this may scramble the egg.

3 Massage half the shampoo mixture into the hair and scalp and rinse well with water. Apply the remaining mixture and leave on the hair for a few minutes before rinsing out thoroughly with warm water.

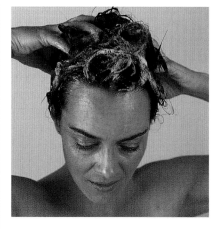

Frequent-use shampoo

The addition of camomile makes this a favourite for regular shampooing.

INGREDIENTS

4 teabags of camomile tea or one handful
   camomile flowers
350ml/12fl oz/1½ cups boiling water
60ml/4 tbsp soap flakes
30ml/2 tbsp honey

1 Steep the teabags or flowers in the boiling water for 10 minutes.

2 Strain the liquid into a bowl and stir in the soap flakes and honey. Cool.

3 Wet the hair, then massage half of the mixture into the scalp and hair. Rinse.

HAIR TIPS

Always use a shampoo that suits your hair and before washing the hair, brush it well to remove any tangles and loosen dirt and skin cells. Rinse your hair with lukewarm water.

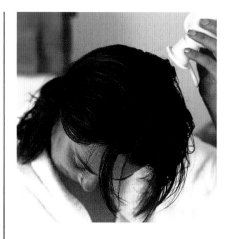

Anti-dandruff shampoo

To make an anti-dandruff shampoo, use a mixture of rosemary and honey. If you like, massage a little liquid into the scalp before bedtime in-between shampoos.

INGREDIENTS

5ml/1 tsp dried rosemary
5ml/1 tsp dried thyme
150ml/¼ pint/⅔ cup boiling water
15ml/1 tbsp honey
150ml/¼ pint/⅔ cup cider vinegar

1 Place the herbs in a bowl and pour over the boiling water.

2 Add the honey and mix until it is melted. Cover and allow to steep for 20 minutes.

3 Strain the mixture into a bottle or jar.

4 Add the cider vinegar and shake well to mix.

5 Wet the hair and massage in some of the shampoo. Rinse. Store the remaining shampoo in a cool, dry place.

Conditioner

Once you have made your chosen shampoo, you may need a conditioner to complete your haircare routine, particularly if your hair is dry, fine or coloured. The hair follicles need natural vitamins and minerals to feed off and if these are lacking from your diet the condition of your hair will suffer. In medieval times, honey was thought to cure baldness. This may be a little optimistic but honey definitely helps to promote the condition and manageabiity of the hair and scalp.

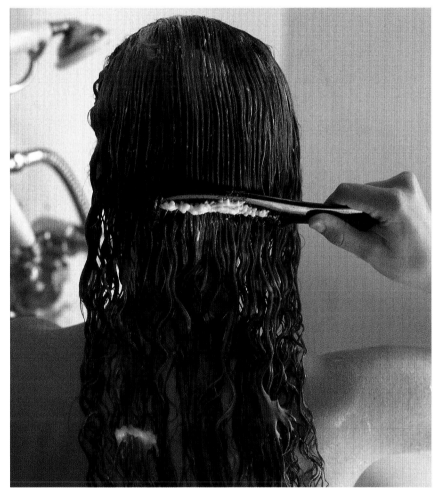

INGREDIENTS

5ml/1 tsp honey

1 egg

10ml/2 tsp coconut or olive oil

1 In a plastic bowl or jug, mix together all the ingredients until blended.

2 Massage over the whole of the scalp. Wrap the head in a warm towel and leave for 30 minutes.

3 Rinse off, then shampoo as normal using a mild shampoo.

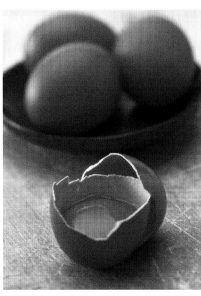

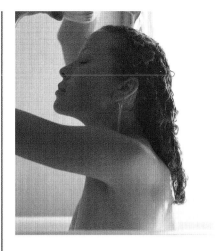

Honey and vinegar rinse

If your hair is in reasonably good condition but just lacks shine, give it a lift with this honey and vinegar rinse.

INGREDIENTS

5ml/1 tsp honey

1 litre/1³⁄₄ pints/4 cups hot water

5ml/1 tsp cider vinegar or lemon juice

1 Mix the ingredients together. Cool.

2 Pour over the hair as a final rinse.

HAIR RINSES

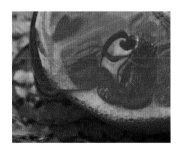

After a honey shampoo, you can enhance your natural hair colour. Sunshine can have a fading effect on the hair, and you may wish to use natural additives in the final rinse of your haircare routine.

For medium brown to dark hair, add cider vinegar to the rinse; for fair to medium fair hair, use lemon juice. Add 25ml/1¹⁄₂ tbsp of cider vinegar or lemon or lime juice to 200ml/7fl oz/scant 1 cup water. Use the mixture as the final rinse.

HONEY FOR NATURAL SKIN TREATMENTS

Honey is the perfect ingredient to add to skin creams because it keeps the skin hydrated and fresh and stops it drying out. Because it is an antimicrobial agent, it also keeps the skin healthy.

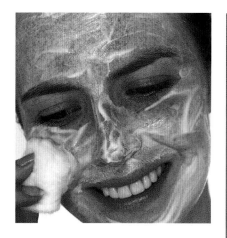

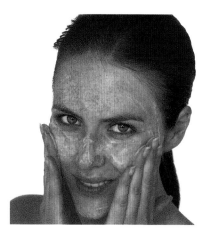

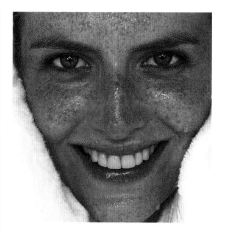

Cleanser

Rosemary and beeswax cream is excellent for removing makeup and mascara and is suitable for most skin types. Make in small quantities and keep for up to one month in the refrigerator.

INGREDIENTS

12g/$\frac{1}{3}$oz beeswax

15g/$\frac{1}{2}$oz emulsifying wax

15ml/1 tbsp coconut oil

100ml/3$\frac{1}{2}$fl oz/scant $\frac{1}{2}$ cup olive oil

1.5ml/$\frac{1}{4}$ tsp borax

30ml/2 tbsp warm water

7.5ml/$\frac{1}{2}$ tbsp rosewater

5 drops rosemary essential oil

1 Melt the beeswax, emulsifying wax, coconut oil and olive oil in a bain marie or microwave.

2 In a separate bowl, dissolve the borax in the warm water.

3 Slowly add the melted oils from the first bowl, stirring constantly. When lukewarm, add the oil and rosewater. When cool, refrigerate.

Facial scrub

Using a scrub is a great way of exfoliating dead skin cells on the face and attacking oily areas where blackheads and blemishes occur. There are many varieties of ingredients that you can use to achieve this and you can have fun trying out your own versions of this base recipe. The honey and banana are rich rehydrators to counteract the abrasiveness of the scrub and will also give a scrumptious fragrance to the mix.

INGREDIENTS

120ml/4fl oz/$\frac{1}{2}$ cup oatmeal, coffee grains or sugar granules

30ml/2 tbsp honey

1 ripe banana

1 Mix all the ingredients together to form a thick paste.

2 Massage over the face, focusing on areas that need attention and avoiding the eyes. Leave on for a few minutes before washing off with a soft cloth and warm water, followed by a splash of astringent.

Skin tonic

The old remedy of placing a slice of cucumber over each eye to reduce any puffiness and refresh tired eyes has a new twist. Pollen promotes the healing of damaged skin, so if your skin looks a bit sluggish, a cucumber tonic is an instant brightener. The vitamin C in cucumber improves circulation, clarity and texture, leaving the skin luminous.

INGREDIENTS

$\frac{1}{2}$ cucumber

30ml/2 tbsp pollen granules

30ml/2 tbsp natural (plain) yogurt (optional)

1 Cut the cucumber into chunks and add the pollen granules. Mash together or whizz in a liquidizer.

2 Strain before use.

3 If you want a thicker preparation, add the natural yogurt.

4 Decant the mixture to a previously sterilized container and when cold, refrigerate until ready to use.

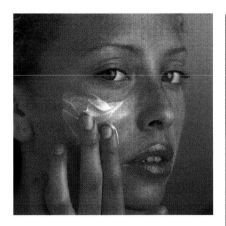

Face moisturizer

All lotions and creams have three main components – water, oil and an emulsifying agent that encourages the water and oil to combine. This cream contains rosewater and almond oil and the emulsifier is beeswax. Honey is added because of its moisturizing qualities and its ability to hold moisture. Essential oils are added to give a light fragrance to the cream and the addition of vitamin E oil is effective in ironing out wrinkles and fading scars on the skin.

INGREDIENTS

10g/¼oz beeswax

20ml/4 tsp almond oil

75ml/5 tbsp rosewater or distilled water

10ml/2 tsp honey

few drops of frankincense, geranium or rose absolute essential oils (optional)

1 vitamin E capsule (optional)

1 Heat together the beeswax and oil in a bain marie or microwave until the wax is just melted.

2 Heat together the water and honey until just under boiling. Combine with the beeswax mixture and mix together for 5 minutes.

3 Set aside until lukewarm, then add any optional ingredients. Pour into a wide-necked jar and when cool, put a lid on and store in the refrigerator.

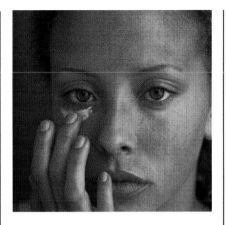

Eye cream

Honey's ability to attract and seal in moisture is put to use in this eye cream, which leaves skin soft and supple. Make a fresh formula for each application, then gently pat the mixture on to the tissue around the eyes, avoiding dragging the skin. Once dry, remove gently by washing off with warm water. For more mature skin, add frankincense essential oil, known for its anti-ageing properties. Apply with care, making sure that you keep the mixture away from the eye directly, working only on the surrounding areas.

INGREDIENTS

15ml/1 tbsp honey

1 egg white

3–5 drops frankincense essential oil (optional)

1 Mix the honey with the egg white.

2 Add the essential oil, if using, and mix.

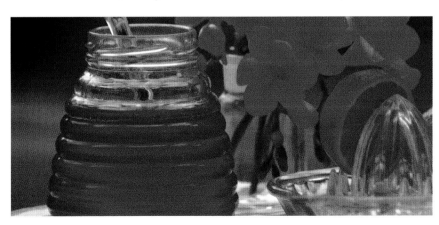

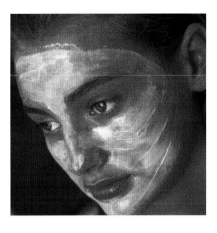

Mask

Face masks are great to help soften and clean the skin, and honey on its own or blended with a little rosewater makes a very basic mask. Manuka honey is expensive but it has excellent healing properties and is ideal for treating skin conditions. Before applying the mask, wash your face in warm water to open the pores. Spread the mask on your face, avoiding the eyes, and leave for 15–30 minutes. Wash off with a soft flannel. To make a more substantial mask, add oatmeal to the mix. Using this once a week will leave you with glowing skin.

INGREDIENTS

50g/2oz/1 cup oatmeal

30ml/1 tbsp honey

5ml/1 tsp rosewater

1 Blend the oatmeal with the honey and add the rosewater.

2 Mix until a smooth paste is formed.

HONEY FOR HAND AND NAIL CARE

Honey is one of the finest skin foods so it is often used as an ingredient in hand cream or barrier cream. It helps hands exposed to harsh weather conditions and water.

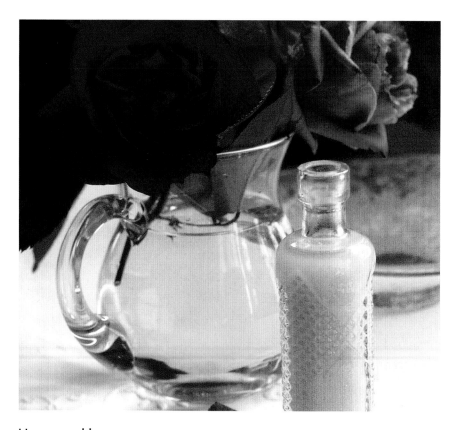

Honey and beeswax cream

The hands are very noticeable because they are always on show, and they age quickly owing to exposure to the elements. Because they are being frequently immersed in water and harsh detergents, the skin dries out faster than on other areas of the body.

Other factors such as heating and air conditioning also have a drying effect. Rough skin and premature aging can be arrested by a daily application of a cream containing honey and beeswax. The honey helps to nourish the hands and slows down the aging process, while beeswax is a good emollient and makes an excellent barrier, so that water, which dries out the hands, cannot penetrate the skin.

INGREDIENTS

10ml/2 tsp beeswax granules

30ml/2 tbsp honey

10ml/2 tsp olive oil

10 drops rose essential oil

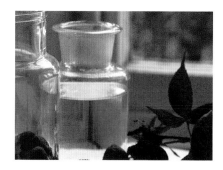

1 Warm the beeswax granules in a bain marie until melted. Put in a bottle or flask and add the honey, olive oil and rose essential oil. Shake the bottle well to mix.

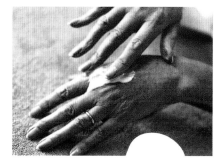

2 Shake the bottle until the cream is smooth, then apply to the hands. If using it at night, wear either cotton or latex gloves overnight. The next day, rub in any cream that remains.

HANDY TIPS

• Always rub in hand cream after a bath or washing your hands, while the skin is still warm, so that it will sink in easily.

• Keep a bottle of hand cream near to the sink to remind you to use it after washing up. Have another bottle next to your bed so you can apply cream before you go to sleep.

• To quickly exfoliate your hands, mix some sea salt and lemon juice together, rub into the hands and rinse off. This will remove dead skin cells and soften skin.

• For a 5-minute treatment, mix 5ml/1 tsp olive oil with 5ml/1 tsp honey. Rub over the hands so they are coated with a thin layer, then wear latex gloves with cotton gloves on top. Leave overnight to allow the skin to absorb the treatment.

• To stimulate circulation, rub the palm of one hand over the back of the other hand.

Cuticle softener

The cuticle is the protective layer of skin at the base of the finger or toe nail that often becomes dry and ragged as it builds up. Never cut the cuticles because they are sealed barriers that prevent infection. To make it easier to push back or remove during regular nailcare, a softener is often applied. Using a natural product containing honey has the added benefit of fighting any build up of bacteria and nourishing the nail itself. Use regularly by massaging the mixture into the cuticles and leave for a few minutes. If you want to have a more intense treatment, leave the cuticle softener on overnight and sleep in a pair of cotton gloves.

INGREDIENTS

1 lemon

5ml/1 tsp honey

5ml/1 tsp almond oil

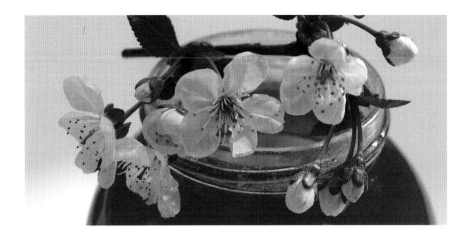

NAIL TIPS

• When filing your nails, prevent them splitting by filing them into a square or oval shape. Don't file them low into the corners because this can weaken the nails. File gently in one long stroke, from the side to the centre of the nail. The best length for nails is just over the fingertip.

• Exposure to water causes nails to become soft and to damage easily, so wear latex gloves when washing dishes to protect your nails.

• Before gardening, drag your nails over a bar of soap because when the nails are full of the soap, there is no space for dirt. The soap can be gently scraped out when you are finished.

• Don't file your nails after a bath when they are soft and pliable or they are likely to split.

• Buff the nails once a week: any more and it will weaken them.

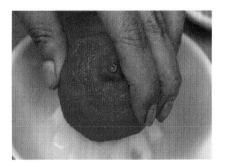

1 Squeeze the lemon and transfer 5ml/ 1 tsp juice to a small bowl.

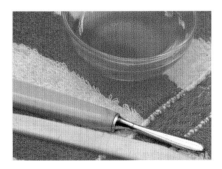

2 Add the honey and almond oil to the lemon juice.

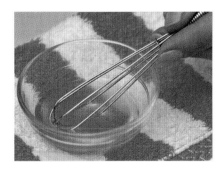

3 Whisk the ingredients until thoroughly blended together.

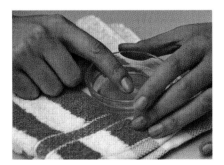

4 Dip each finger into the mixture. Leave for a few seconds.

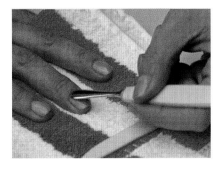

5 Using a cuticle tool, push down on the cuticles very gently.

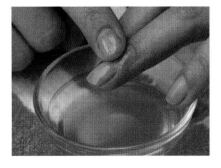

6 Massage into the nails using a circular movement until absorbed.

HONEY FOR LIPS

For the nourishing and healing of dry or chapped lips, particularly in the winter months, this balm made with beeswax and essential oil has a rich emollient effect.

It is simple to make your own lip balm to moisturize and soothe lips that have been affected by the sun and the wind, the temperature or even by illness. This balm is very easy to make and contains honey and beeswax, which are excellent for moisturizers. For a simple instant balm, just combine a drop of honey with a flavouring such as vanilla or rosewater. Either will make a quick salve for sore or chapped lips.

If your lips are flaking, gently remove any dead skin with a soft toothbrush, then apply the lip balm. Another method is to coat the lips with petroleum jelly. Leave it to work for a few minutes, then gently rub your lips with a warm damp cloth. The flakes of skin will be removed.

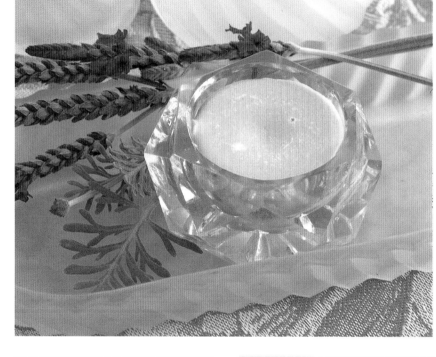

INGREDIENTS

30ml/2 tbsp coconut or olive oil

15ml/1 tbsp beeswax

4 drops lavender, lemon or
   peppermint essential oil

vitamin E capsule or equivalent in
   vitamin E oil

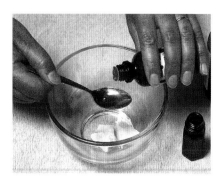

1 Mix the coconut oil, beeswax and essential oil in a bowl. Place in a bain marie, or in a pan of simmering water.

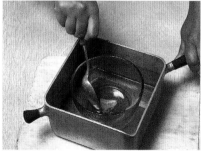

2 Blend the ingredients gently together with a spoon or spatula until the wax is completely melted.

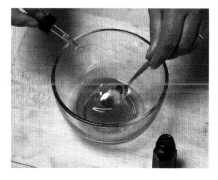

TIPS FOR USING BEESWAX

• Beeswax melts at 147°C/64°F and should not be overheated because it then loses its aroma and becomes very brittle and liable to develop cracks when cooled.

• Beeswax is very inflammable, so always melt it in a bain marie or in a microwave, but never melt it in a pan over a flame.

• It takes about 45 seconds to melt beeswax in a microwave and 3 minutes in a bain marie.

3 Break open the vitamin E capsule, add the contents to the wax mixture and mix well. Pour the mixture into a suitable container and allow to cool and set.

HONEY FOR FRESH BREATH

Sometimes cleaning your teeth is not enough and a gargle with a mouthwash with antiseptic and antibacterial properties is needed to help fight any plaque-forming bacteria.

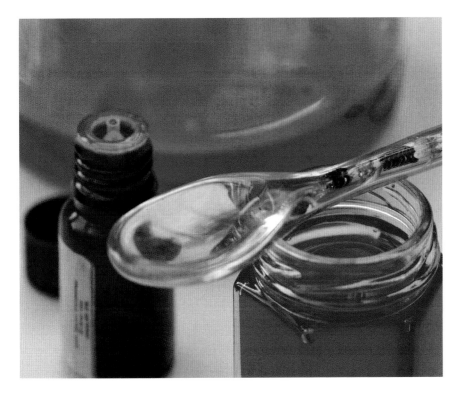

Often a mouth rinse is necessary for good oral hygiene. This excellent mouthwash is simply made with ingredients from your storecupboard. It is easily prepared if you would like a change from your usual product or if you prefer a natural option that is free of chemicals. Honey is a well-known antibacterial agent, as well as having antiseptic properties, so it is a perfect addition to this mouthwash. It is known that its bactericide (bacteria-killing) properties increase when diluted with water. Store in a cool place and use to rinse your mouth every morning and evening, or after you brush your teeth.

INGREDIENTS

5ml/1 tsp dried peppermint or
 dried spearmint
5ml/1 tsp dried thyme
5ml/1 tsp crushed cloves
500ml/17fl oz/generous 2 cups distilled
 water or cider vinegar
5ml/1 tsp honey
10 drops peppermint essential oil

HONEY AS AN ANTIBACTERIAL AGENT

• Honey inhibits bacterial action and thus blocks oral bacteria.

• When added to a mouthwash, honey kills germs in the mouth and cleans teeth and dentures.

• As well as freshening breath, honey helps to heal mouth ulcers.

• When used regularly, honey mouthwash will help to heal any sores in the mouth.

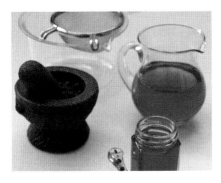

1 Mix the peppermint, dried thyme and crushed cloves with the water or cider vinegar. Soak for 7–10 days.

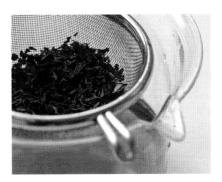

2 Strain the mixture through a sieve and reserve the liquid in a bowl. Discard the dried herbs.

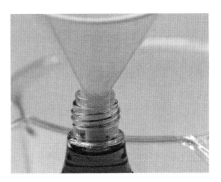

3 Add the honey and the peppermint oil. Pour the mouthwash into a clean bottle or jar, ready for use.

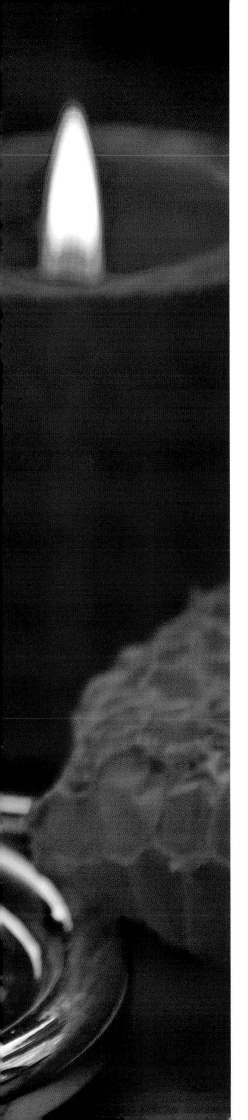

HONEY AND BEESWAX IN THE HOUSE AND GARDEN

Beeswax is an ingredient in many common household products – candles, soaps and furniture polishes. It is used to make candles because it burns cleanly with no residue and minimal smoke; in polish it provides a smooth and protective finish for wood, and it can even be used for lubricating drawer runners and racquet handles. Soap, hand cream, bath oils and bath lotions sometimes contain beeswax because it is so softening and soothing to the skin.

Left: Candles made from beeswax burn brighter, cleaner and longer than any other type of wax candles – and they smell good too.

USING BEE PRODUCTS IN THE HOME

Beeswax and honey have been used around the house since ancient times and because they are natural products without any toxic or artificial additives, they are still popular today.

Both honey and beeswax are found together in some household products, such as soaps, while beeswax is used alone in good quality candles and polishes for wood and leather.

Soap, candles and polishes

Beeswax and honey are popular ingredients in home-made soaps because of the emollient qualities of beeswax and its ability to form a barrier to protect the skin. The addition of beeswax to home-made soap makes a hard, creamy soap with an aromatic scent that does not contain any harmful synthetic ingredients, and it is mild enough for even the most sensitive skin.

Candles made from beeswax are popular in the home because they burn brighter, hotter and longer than candles made from paraffin wax. Also, they have the advantage of being smokeless, and they do not drip. Beeswax candles create a relaxing atmosphere because they release a sweet aromatic scent that is derived from the honey and pollen that remain in the honeycomb cells.

Beeswax polishes have traditionally been used in the home to either revive distressed wood or leather, or to enhance the fine patina of wooden furniture, as well as impart a wonderfully silky, protective finish. In addition, the polish is natural with no harsh chemicals to harm the environment, and has a pleasant aroma with a hint of honey.

Small wooden balls polished with honey or beeswax can be used in closets and drawers to deter moths and to add a honeyed scent to your clothes.

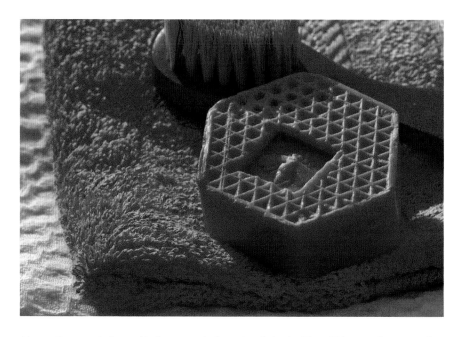

Above: Beeswax is formed in hexagonal-shaped cells in the hive. Older wax is removed and is used in the manufacture of products such as soap.

Honey and beeswax will add subtle fragrance to your home, and help to enhance your health and wellbeing.

Christmas tree reviver

An unusual use of honey is for reviving and freshening a Christmas tree that is required to last through the holiday season. If the tree has no roots and you want to check the freshness of the tree, simply rub your finger over the base. If your finger feels slightly sticky, there is still sap on the stump, indicating that it has been freshly cut. If not, you can make a solution that mimics the sap of a live tree by mixing 250ml/8fl oz/1 cup honey and 200g/7oz sugar with 10 litres/2.6 gallons water. Stir well, then pour the mixture into a bucket and stand the tree in it. This treatment helps to keep the tree perky and reduces the rate of pine needles falling off throughout the Christmas festivities.

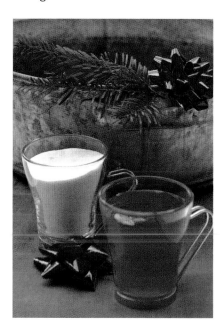

Right: Stand your Christmas tree in a honey mixture to keep it looking festive.

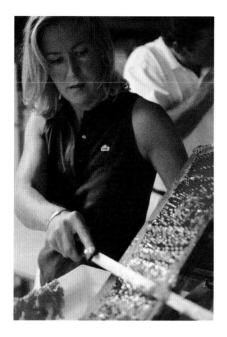

Above: A woman is trimming the wax cappings from a large hive frame to release the honey that is sealed beneath.

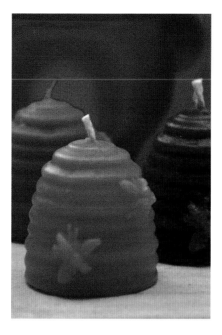

Above: Beeswax candles are said to be the finest because they burn brighter, hotter and cleaner than other candles.

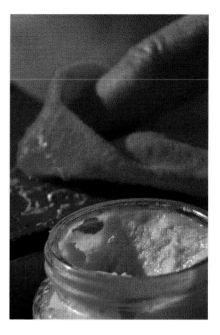

Above: Beeswax polish gives a smooth and shiny finish to wooden furniture and has a lovely honey aroma.

GOLF CLUB GRIP WAX

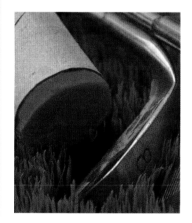

Most golfers need to regrip their clubs once a year. For the occasional golfer, this can be extended by several months with regular maintenance. Waxing will prevent grips becoming slippery or cracked and improve the golfer's grip in wet conditions.

To make the grip wax, melt 50g/2oz beeswax with 5ml/1 tsp powdered resin in a bain marie. Meanwhile, create a 10cm/4in diameter tube from thick paper, or use a cardboard tube. Fill the tube with the melted mixture. Once set, use to wax the grip of golf clubs or tennis racquets, peeling the paper away as the wax is used.

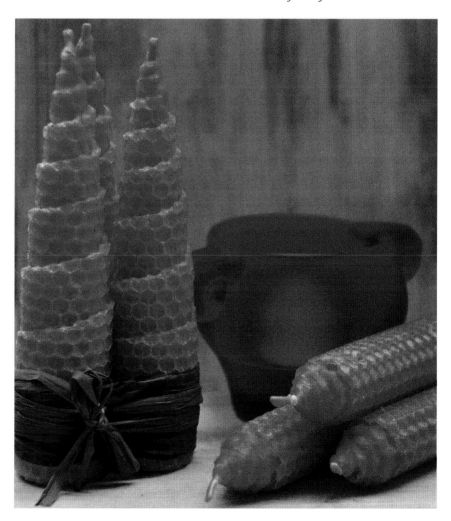

Above: Sheets of beeswax can be rolled into straight candles or spiral-shaped candles. Because they produce negative ions while burning, they leave the air fresher and cleaner.

BEESWAX POLISHES

Beeswax polish not only has a fragrant scent, it imparts a wonderful shine to leather and wooden furniture, and it is very simple to make your own regular supply at home.

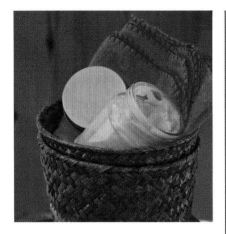

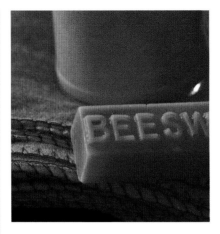

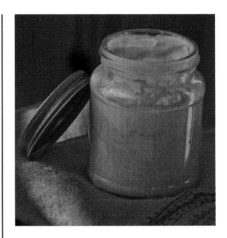

Solid furniture polish

Start by making small quantities. For a soft satin shine on wood, substitute carnauba wax for the linseed oil and increase the turpentine by 100ml/3½fl oz/½ cup.

INGREDIENTS

175g/6oz/1½ cups beeswax

250ml/8fl oz/1 cup linseed oil

250ml/8fl oz/1 cup turpentine

1 Using a microwave or bain marie, warm the beeswax, linseed oil and turpentine. Mix well off the heat.

2 Pour the polish into a clean jar with a wide neck and allow to set. Apply to the item, dry and buff with a soft cloth. For best results, rub in small circles.

REMOVING BEESWAX FROM FURNITURE

If beeswax is accidentally spilled on a wooden surface, take off as much as possible, then heat the area using a hair dryer on a low setting. Once the wax liquifies, wipe clean with a dry cloth.

Liquid polish

For those who prefer a liquid polish, this one includes liquid paraffin.

INGREDIENTS

50g/2oz/½ cup beeswax

30ml/2 tbsp carnauba wax

550ml/18fl oz/2½ cups liquid paraffin

1 Using a microwave or bain marie, melt the waxes. Remove from the heat.

2 Stir in the liquid paraffin.

Cream polish

INGREDIENTS

50ml/2fl oz/¼ cup liquid soap

250ml/8fl oz/1 cup water

75g/3oz/5 tbsp beeswax

500ml/17fl oz/generous 2 cups turpentine

50ml/2fl oz/¼ cup pine oil

1 Heat the soap and water. In a bain marie, melt the beeswax and add the turpentine and pine oil.

2 When each mix is cool, mix together.

Leather treatment

To waterproof leather, nourish and stop it cracking, prepare the treatment below and, while still warm, apply with a dry cloth, or, brush it on to the leather. Polish with a clean dry cloth.

INGREDIENTS

50g/2oz/½ cup beeswax

50g/2oz/½ cup resin

600ml/1 pint/2½ cups vegetable oil

1 Using a microwave or bain marie, gently melt the beeswax.

2 Add the resin and oil. Stir well to mix.

REMOVING BEESWAX FROM A CARPET

To remove beeswax from carpet and upholstery, take off as much beeswax as possible by hand, then place a piece of kitchen or brown paper over the area. Apply a warm iron, moving over the wax as it soaks into the paper. Apply with care, as some fabrics may be too delicate for this treatment.

BEESWAX AND HONEY SOAP

Containing both beeswax and honey, this soap has an aromatic fragance and a moisturizing texture. Add flowers or herbs if you wish, or oatmeal for an exfoliating effect.

This mixture sets quickly, so any added ingredients, including essential oils for fragrance, colouring and solids, such as pot pourri, herbs or oatmeal, need to be at the ready. The best colourings for soap are from spices and plants, such as turmeric if you want a yellow colour. Experiment with moulds; there are many things around the house that can be used to make interesting soap bars, such as plastic pastry cutters, small bowls or cups. Muffin moulds can make great soap-on-ropes if a looped piece of cord is held upright in the centre of the mould while the liquid is poured around it.

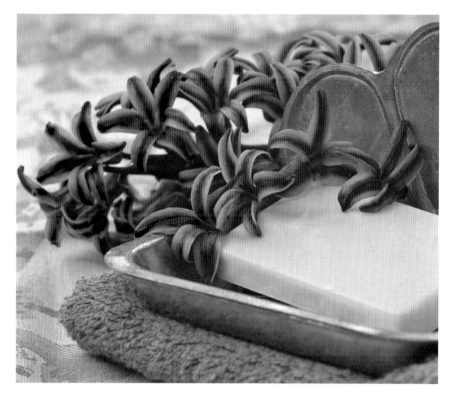

INGREDIENTS

25g/1oz/¼ cup beeswax

50g/2oz/1 cup lye

250ml/8fl oz/1 cup cold water

450ml/¾ pint/scant 2 cups olive oil

25ml/1½ tbsp honey

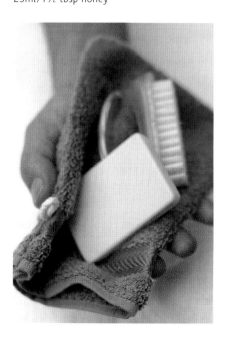

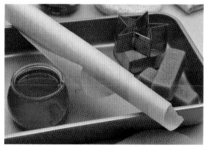

1 Assemble all the ingredients. Place the beeswax in a heatproof bowl, then melt in a bain marie or microwave.

2 Heat the lye with the water in a pan. Add the olive oil, gently heat, then add to the beeswax. Stir until the mixture is blended and the water has evaporated.

3 Pour the mixture into plastic moulds and cover with greaseproof paper. Leave aside to cool for 48 hours. After cooling, place the moulds in the freezer for about 2 hours. This makes it easier to remove the soap from the moulds.

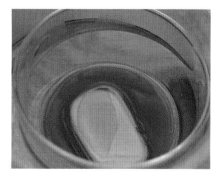

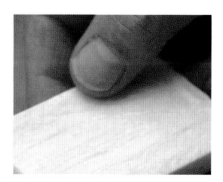

COLD PROCESS CANDLES

For a speedy sophisticated candle, ready-prepared beeswax sheets are simply rolled up with a wick in the middle to produce a fine candle that burns with a delicate aroma.

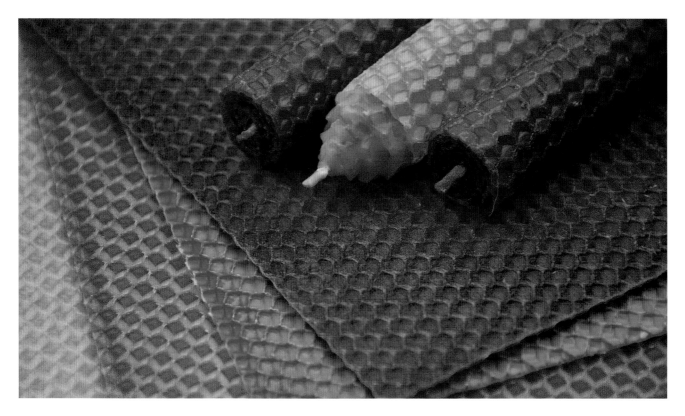

INGREDIENTS

sheets of beeswax

cotton wick

1 For a tapered candle, warm some sheets of beeswax with a hairdryer to keep them malleable. The short side of the sheet will determine the height of the candle. Using a craft knife, cut a narrow triangular segment off the longest side.

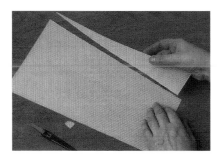

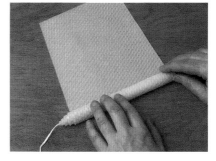

2▲ Cut a wick that will extend about 2cm/³⁄₄in above the height of the candle. Press the wick along the shorter side and roll up. Check that the wick is being held closely from the first turn.

3➤ When you have finished rolling the wax, press the edge into the candle to give a smooth finish. Trim the wick, then wrap a tiny piece of wax around it so that it is primed and ready for burning.

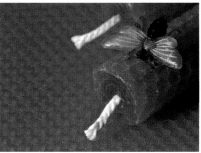

Above: Using sheets of beeswax, you can make candles of the length and width that you prefer.

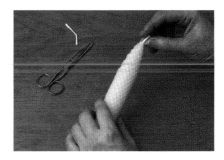

HOT PROCESS CANDLES

It's fun to make candles at home. You can make basic, traditional dipped candles or use moulds lined with shells or dried herbs to create more stylish candles.

INGREDIENTS

450g/1lb beeswax

colouring (wax crayon or pigment)

25ml/1½ tbsp essential oil (optional)

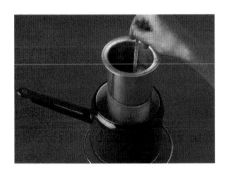

1 Melt the wax in a bain marie or microwave; you can put the wax in a can and stand it in a saucepan of water. Heat the water to melt the wax, stirring occasionally. Test the temperature of the water with a thermometer. When the temperature is approximately 71°C/160°F, turn down the heat. Stir to avoid air bubbles in the wax.

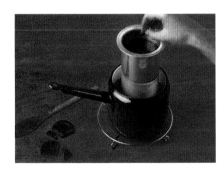

2 To colour the wax, add small pieces of solid dye, stirring well so that the wax and dye are well blended. Take care not to add too much dye because the colour is very intense. If you wish to add fragrance, add the essential oil of your choice. Stir for 2 minutes to mix thoroughly.

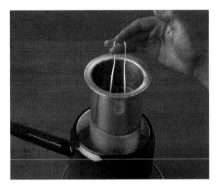

3 Check that the temperature has not dropped; if it has bring it back to 71°C/160°F. Prime the wick by dipping it in the melted wax until it is sealed. Leave to cool, then hang them over a rail. Repeat the dipping and drying processes until the candles are the size you require; this will take 15–30 dips.

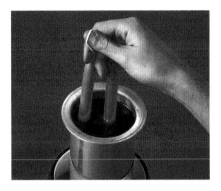

4 To give the candles a smooth outer surface, increase the heat of the wax to 82°C/180°F, then dip the candles in the wax for about 3 seconds and leave to cool. When they are cool, trim the bases with a knife until they are flat. Leave the finished candles to cool for at least 1 hour before burning.

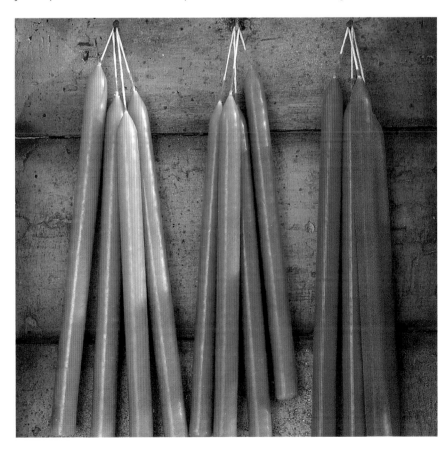

WAX CRAYONS

Crayons made with beeswax are sturdy and easy for children to handle and use for drawing and colouring activities. The use of beeswax allows the pigment to shine through.

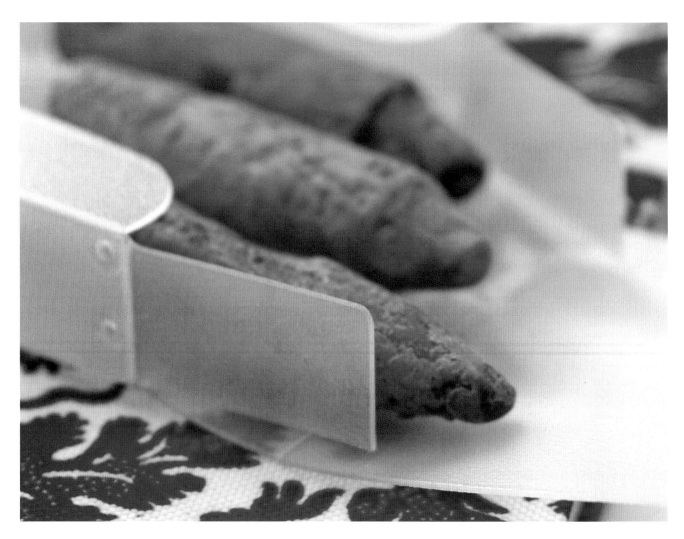

INGREDIENTS

2 parts beeswax

1 part talc

artist's pigment or food colouring

aluminium foil, rolled up for moulds, one end
  twisted to seal

oil, for brushing

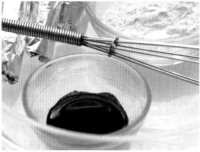

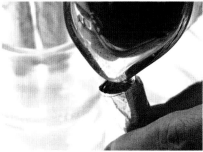

1 Melt the beeswax either in a microwave or in a bain marie. Once liquified, add the talc and then the colouring bit by bit until it reaches the density of colour required.

2 Very carefully pour the hot mixture into the moulds and leave to set. When the wax is beginning to set but is still malleable, gently shape a point at the end of each crayon. Leave until hard.

HONEY FLY TRAP

This simple device for catching flies has even been used by armies on manoeuvre. It is a fairly unusual use of honey, but needs only basic ingredients that you will have in the home.

INGREDIENTS

a large plastic bottle

knife

100ml/3½fl oz/scant ½ cup each of honey
   and water

strong waterproof adhesive tape

60cm/24in of thin string

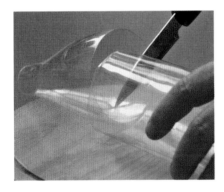

1 Dampen the label from the plastic bottle and remove it. Rinse out with water and discard the cap. Use the knife to neatly cut the bottle in half.

2 Add the honey and water to a jug and stir thoroughly.

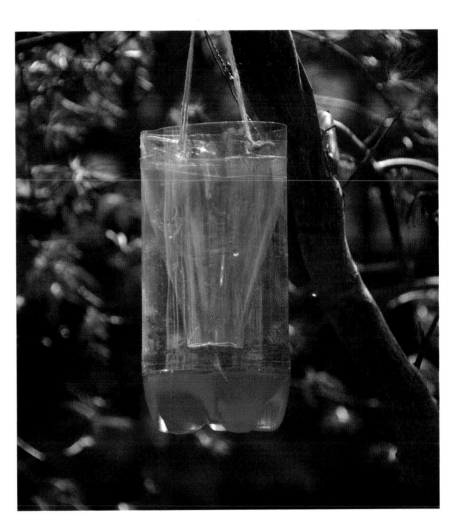

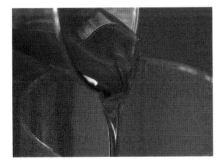

3 Pour the honey mixture into the bottom half of the bottle. Invert the top half of the bottle into the bottom part of the bottle so that the neck of the bottle faces downwards. To prevent flies drowning, use paper to screen the liquid.

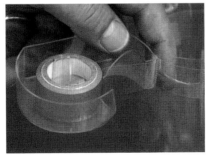

4 Tape the two halves of the bottle together, using a strong waterproof adhesive tape. Wind the tape around twice to ensure that the structure holds together when it is hung up. Replenish the mixture when required.

HANGING TRAP

If you want to hang the trap in the garden so that it does not entice rodents, create a hanger as follows. On opposite sides of the container, make two holes, lace 60cm/24in of string through the holes and tie with a secure knot, then hang it up.

A simpler version of this trap simply requires the string to be dipped into pure honey and pinned up wherever required. The flies will stick to the honey and when covered, the string can bagged for disposal.

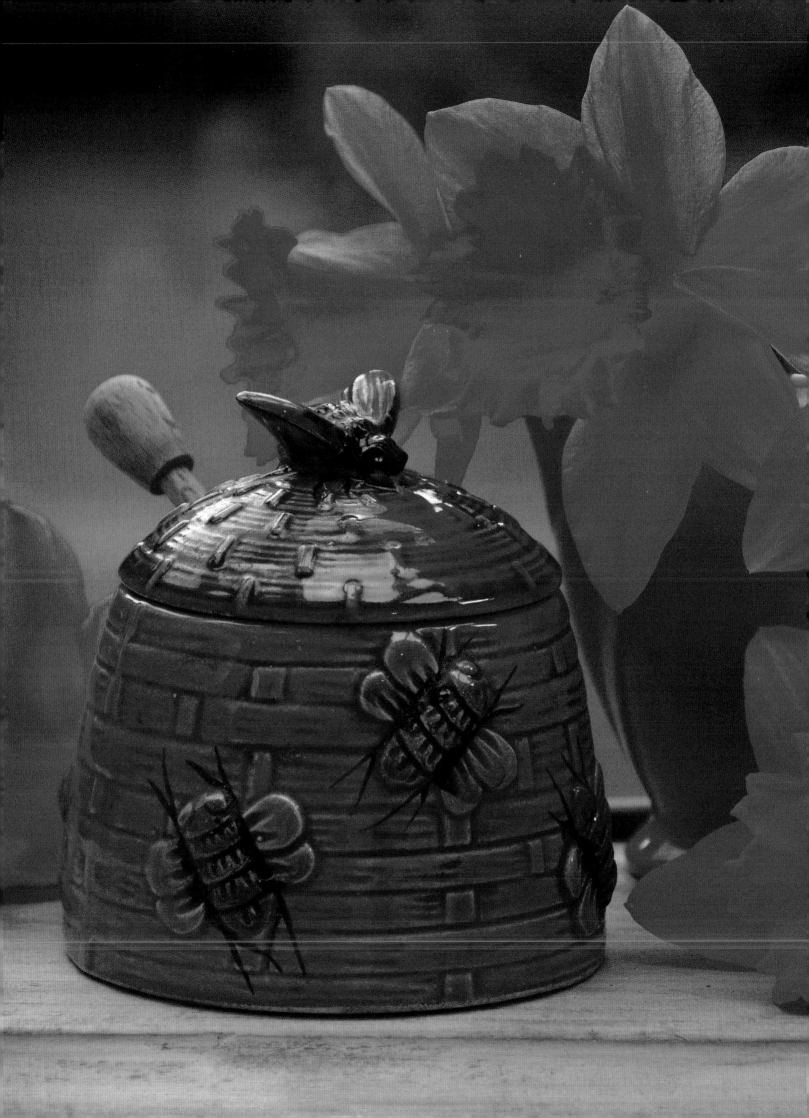

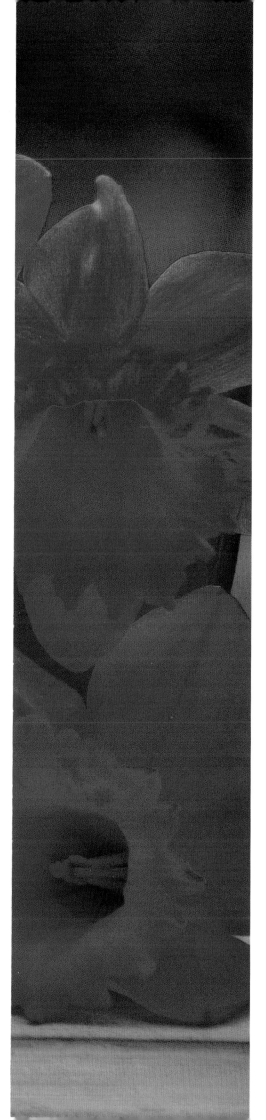

HONEY IN THE KITCHEN

The oldest sweetener known to man, honey fell out of favour somewhat when cane and beet sugar came on the scene. In recent years it has made a big comeback, however. This is partly because of growing interest in organic foods and partly because more and more people are discovering the versatility of honey and the subtle variations in flavour offered by the different types. Also, unlike sugar, honey has the property of absorbing moisture, so baked foods will stay fresh and moist longer.

Left: The bee motif is a popular one for kitchen china.

HONEY WITH MEAT

Honey enhances any meat and robustly stands up to spices, herbs and chillies. Lamb, pork and beef dishes all benefit from the addition of honey.

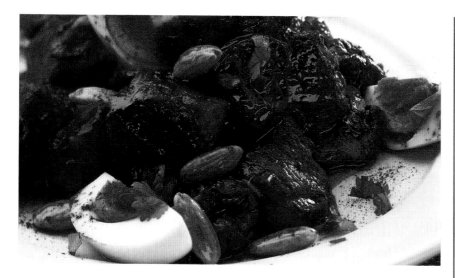

Lamb with honey and prunes
INGREDIENTS

Serves 6

130g/4½oz/generous ½ cup pitted prunes
350ml/12fl oz/1½ cups hot tea
1kg/2¼lb stewing lamb, cut into chunks
1 onion, chopped
75–90ml/5–6 tbsp chopped fresh parsley
2.5ml/½ tsp ground ginger
2.5ml/½ tsp curry powder
pinch of grated fresh nutmeg
10ml/2 tsp ground cinnamon
1.5ml/¼ tsp saffron threads
75–120ml/5–9 tbsp honey, to taste
250ml/8fl oz/1 cup beef or lamb stock
115g/4oz/1 cup blanched almonds, toasted
30ml/2 tbsp chopped fresh coriander
  (cilantro) leaves
3 hard-boiled eggs, cut into wedges
salt and ground black pepper

1 Preheat the oven to 180°C/350°F/ Gas 4. Put the prunes in a bowl, pour over the hot tea and leave to soak up the tea and plump up.

2 Meanwhile, put the lamb into a roasting pan with the onion, parsley, ginger, curry powder, nutmeg, cinnamon, the salt and a large pinch of ground black pepper. Cover the roasting pan and cook in the preheated oven for about 2 hours, or until the meat is just tender.

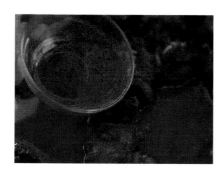

3 Drain the prunes and add their liquid to the lamb. Combine the saffron and 30ml/2 tbsp hot water and add to the pan with the honey and stock. Bake, uncovered, for 30 minutes, turning occasionally. Add the prunes and serve with the almonds, coriander and egg.

Energy 618Kcal/2,564kJ; **Protein** 42.7g; **Carbohydrate** 0.8g, of which sugars 0.1g; **Fat** 49.3g, of which saturates 21.2g; **Cholesterol** 183mg; **Calcium** 16mg; **Fibre** 0.2g; **Sodium** 150mg.

Minted lamb with honey
INGREDIENTS

Serves 2

30ml/2 tbsp olive oil
15ml/1 tbsp lemon juice
30ml/2 tbsp chopped fresh mint
4 lamb chops or steaks
250g/9oz/2 cups leeks, thinly sliced
1 garlic clove, finely chopped
45ml/3 tbsp double (heavy) cream
15ml/1 tbsp clear honey

1 In a shallow container, mix 15ml/ 1 tbsp of the oil with the lemon juice and 15ml/1 tbsp of the mint. Season. Add the lamb and turn in the mint mixture. Leave in the refrigerator for 30 minutes. Turn the lamb twice.

2 Fry the lamb in the remaining oil. Cook over medium heat for 6–8 minutes each side or until browned. Remove from the pan and keep warm.

3 Drain off most of the excess fat from the pan. Add the leeks and garlic, and scrape up any sediment from the base of the pan. Cover and cook over medium heat for 5 minutes, stirring occasionally, until the leeks are soft.

4 Stir in the remaining mint, cream and honey and heat gently until bubbling. Adjust the seasoning if necessary. Serve the leeks in the sauce with the lamb.

Energy 521Kcal/2,166kJ; **Protein** 31.8g; **Carbohydrate** 7.9g, of which sugars 7g; **Fat** 40.5g, of which saturates 17g; **Cholesterol** 145mg; **Calcium** 54mg; **Fibre** 2.8g; **Sodium** 137mg.

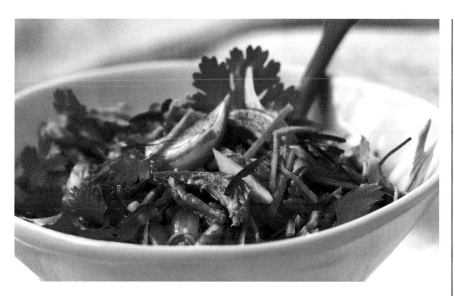

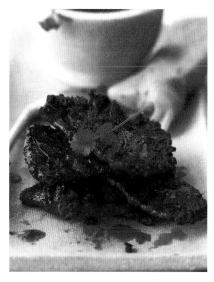

Sweet-and-sour pork with honey
INGREDIENTS

Serves 4

30ml/2 tbsp dark soy sauce

15ml/1 tbsp clear honey

400g/14oz pork fillet (tenderloin)

6 shallots, very thinly sliced lengthways

1 lemon grass stalk, thinly sliced

5 kaffir lime leaves, thinly sliced

5cm/2in piece fresh root ginger, sliced

1/2 fresh long red chilli, seeded and sliced

bunch fresh coriander (cilantro), chopped

For the dressing

30ml/2 tbsp palm sugar

30ml/2 tbsp Thai fish sauce

juice of 2 limes

20ml/4 tsp thick tamarind juice, made by
    mixing tamarind paste with warm water

1 Preheat the grill (broiler). Put the soy sauce and the honey in a small bowl and mix well.

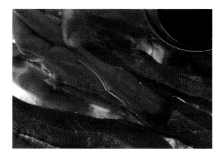

2 Using a sharp knife, cut the pork fillet lengthways into quarters to make four long, thick strips. Place them in a grill (broiling) pan. Brush with the soy sauce and honey mixture, then grill (broil) for about 10–15 minutes, until cooked through. Turn the strips over often and baste with the honey mixture.

3 Transfer the cooked pork strips to a board. Slice the meat across the grain, then shred it with a fork. Place in a large bowl and add the shallot slices, lemon grass, kaffir lime leaves, ginger, chilli and chopped coriander.

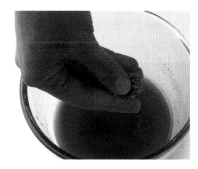

4 Make the dressing. Place the sugar, fish sauce, lime juice and tamarind juice in a bowl. Whisk until the sugar has completely dissolved. Pour the dressing over the pork mixture and toss well to mix, then serve.

Energy 170Kcal/718kJ; **Protein** 22g; **Carbohydrate** 12.2g, of which sugars 12.1g; **Fat** 4g, of which saturates 1.4g; **Cholesterol** 63mg; **Calcium** 16mg; **Fibre** 0.2g; **Sodium** 873mg.

Chilli and honey-cured beef
INGREDIENTS

Serves 4

450g/1lb beef sirloin

2 lemon grass stalks, trimmed and chopped

2 garlic cloves, chopped

2 dried Serrano chillies, seeded and chopped

30–45ml/2–3 tbsp honey

15ml/1 tbsp *nuoc mam* (fish sauce)

30ml/2 tbsp soy sauce

rice wrappers, fresh herbs
    and dipping sauce, to serve (optional)

1 Trim the beef and cut it against the grain into thin, rectangular slices.

2 Using a mortar and pestle, grind the lemon grass, garlic and chillies to a paste. Stir in the honey, nuoc mam and soy sauce. Put the beef into a bowl, tip in the paste and rub it into the meat.

3 Arrange the meat on a rack and put it in the refrigerator, uncovered, for 2 days.

4 Cook the beef on the barbecue and serve as a snack on its own or with rice wrappers, herbs and a dipping sauce.

Energy 138Kcal/581kJ; **Protein** 18g; **Carbohydrate** 9g, of which sugars 8g; **Fat** 3g, of which saturates 2g; **Cholesterol** 38mg; **Calcium** 7mg; **Fibre** 0.1g; **Sodium** 40mg.

HONEY WITH VEGETABLES

Honey brings out the maximum flavour in a range of vegetable dishes, as well as adding a tantalizing hint of sweetness. It also makes a delicious glaze for vegetables.

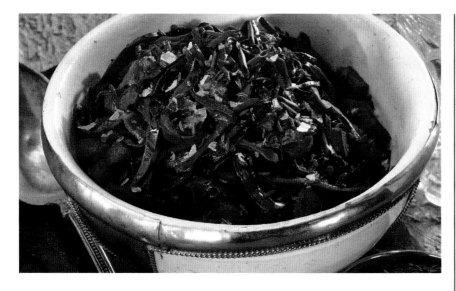

Honeyed red cabbage with spices

INGREDIENTS

Serves 4

3 thick, rindless bacon rashers, diced

1 large onion, chopped

1 large red cabbage, evenly shredded

3 garlic cloves, crushed

15–25ml/1–1½ tbsp caraway
    seeds

120ml/4fl oz/½ cup water

2 firm, ripe pears, peeled,
    cored and chopped

juice of 1 lemon

475ml/16fl oz/2 cups red wine

45ml/3 tbsp red wine vinegar

150g/5oz/scant ¾ cup clear honey

salt and freshly ground black pepper

caraway seeds and snipped fresh chives,
    to garnish

1 Dry fry the bacon over low heat for 5–10 minutes, or until golden brown. Stir in the onion and cook for 5 minutes or until pale golden.

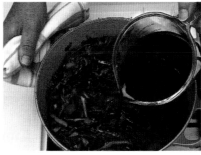

2 Stir the cabbage, garlic, caraway seeds and the water into the pan. Cover and cook for 8–10 minutes. Season, then add the pears, lemon juice, red wine and vinegar. Cover and cook for 15 minutes. Stir in the honey.

3 If there is too much cooking liquid, remove the lid and allow it to reduce. The pears will have broken up in the pot, and the quantity reduced by one-third. Adjust the seasoning to taste and serve sprinkled with caraway seeds and snipped fresh chives.

Energy 112Kcal/469kJ; **Protein** 2g; **Carbohydrate** 17.1g, of which sugars 15.5g; **Fat** 2.4g, of which saturates 1.3g; **Cholesterol** 5mg; **Calcium** 55mg; **Fibre** 3.1g; **Sodium** 25mg.

Honeyed vegetables

INGREDIENTS

Serves 6

250g/9oz carrots, peeled and sliced

1 sweet potato, peeled and cut into chunks

1 potato, peeled and cut into chunks

pinch of sugar

30ml/2 tbsp vegetable oil

1 onion, chopped

10 pitted prunes, halved or quartered

30–45ml/2–3 tbsp currants

5 dried apricots, roughly chopped

30ml/2 tbsp honey

5–10ml/1–2 tsp chopped fresh root ginger

1 cinnamon stick

1 Preheat the oven to 160°C/325°F/ Gas 3. Put the carrots, sweet potato and potato into a pan of sugared and salted boiling water and cook until almost tender. Drain, reserving the cooking liquid, and set aside.

2 Heat the oil in a flameproof casserole, add the onion and fry until softened. Add the cooked vegetables and enough of the cooking liquid to cover the vegetables completely, then add the remaining ingredients.

3 Cover and cook in the oven for 40 minutes. Near the end of cooking time, check the liquid. If there is too much liquid, remove the lid for the last 15 minutes.

Energy 143Kcal/601kJ; **Protein** 1.9g; **Carbohydrate** 26.8g, of which sugars 15.9g; **Fat** 3.9g, of which saturates 2.3g; **Cholesterol** 9mg; **Calcium** 36mg; **Fibre** 2.9g; **Sodium** 55mg.

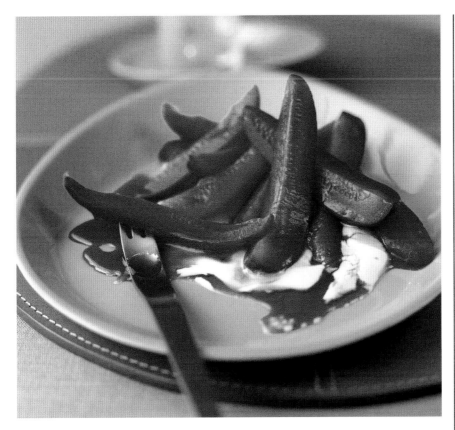

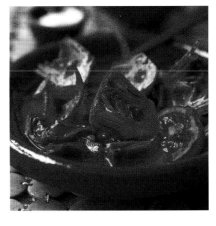

Honey and sour cream gherkins

This salad has Russian origins, and it is traditionally served with a selection of hors d'oeuvres, called zakouski. The honey marries perfectly with the sour cream to give a delightful sweet and sour flavour to the dish. It could act as a perfect foil to grilled or roast pork.

INGREDIENTS

Serves 4

4 large pickled gherkins
60ml/4 tbsp sour cream
15g/$\frac{1}{2}$oz/1 tbsp butter
60ml/4 tbsp clear honey

1 Slice the gherkins lengthways into quarters. Whisk the sour cream until light and foamy, then spoon on to four individual serving plates.

2 Put the butter in a frying pan and heat until melted. Add the gherkin slices and turn in the butter until warmed, then pile on top of the sour cream.

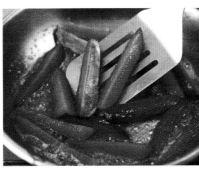

3 Pour the honey into the pan and stir well until all the butter and residue on the bottom of the pan are thoroughly incorporated. Spoon over the gherkins and serve hot.

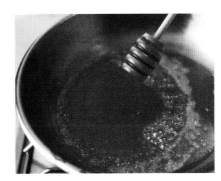

Energy 106Kcal/441kJ; Protein 0.8g; Carbohydrate 12.6g, of which sugars 12.6g; Fat 6.1g, of which saturates 3.8g; Cholesterol 17mg; Calcium 22mg; Fibre 0.2g; Sodium 32mg.

Honeyed artichoke hearts

Globe artichokes are cooked in a honey dressing with ginger and preserved lemons. This dish makes a good accompaniment to barbecued meat.

INGREDIENTS

Serves 4

30–45ml/2–3 tbsp olive oil
2 garlic cloves, crushed
scant 5ml/1 tsp ground ginger
pinch of saffron threads
juice of $\frac{1}{2}$ lemon
15–30ml/1–2 tbsp honey
peel of 1 preserved lemon, finely sliced
8 artichoke hearts, quartered
150ml/$\frac{1}{4}$ pint/$\frac{2}{3}$ cup water
salt

1 Heat the olive oil in a heavy pan and add the garlic. Before the garlic begins to colour, stir in the ginger, saffron, lemon juice, honey and preserved lemon peel. Add the artichokes and toss them in the spices and honey. Add the water and salt and heat until simmering.

2 Cover the pan and simmer for 10–15 minutes. If the liquid has not reduced, take the lid off the pan and boil for 2 minutes until it is reduced to a coating consistency. Serve warm.

Energy 142Kcal/586kJ; Protein 1.6g; Carbohydrate 4.1g, of which sugars 1.9g; Fat 11.3g, of which saturates 1.6g; Cholesterol 0mg; Calcium 40mg; Fibre 1.6g; Sodium 47mg.

HONEY IN DESSERTS

A more obvious use of honey is to sweeten and flavour fruity desserts and ices. Because honey is sweeter than sugar, around one-third less is needed for desserts.

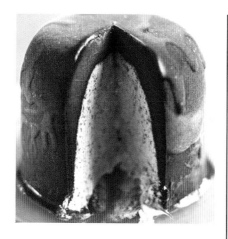

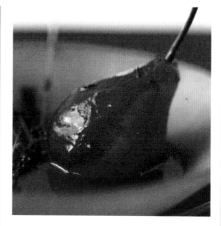

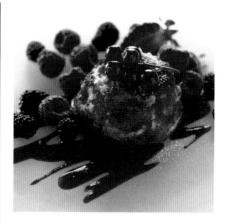

Raspberry and honey bombe
INGREDIENTS
Serves 4

750ml/1¼ pints/3 cups raspberry sorbet
550ml/18fl oz/2½ cups double (heavy) cream
60ml/4 tbsp clear honey
75ml/5 tbsp whisky
50g/2oz/½ cup medium oatmeal, toasted

1 Stand the sorbet at room temperature for 20 minutes. Chill a 1.5 litre/2½ pint/6¼ cup bombe mould. Pack the sorbet on to the base and sides of the mould. Return to the freezer.

2 Whip the cream with the honey and whisky until softly peaking. Fold in the oatmeal. Spoon into the mould and level the surface. Cover and freeze.

3 To serve, loosen the edges of the mould. Dip the mould into hot water, lift out, hold a plate over the top of the mould, then invert on to the plate. Serve.

Energy 518Kcal/2158kJ; **Protein** 3g; **Carbohydrate** 39.2g, of which sugars 34.6g; **Fat** 37.7g, of which saturates 23g; **Cholesterol** 94mg; **Calcium** 68mg; **Fibre** 2.2g; **Sodium** 22mg.

Poached pears in scented honey
INGREDIENTS
Serves 4

45ml/3 tbsp clear honey
juice of 1 lemon
250ml/8fl oz/1 cup water
pinch of saffron threads
1 cinnamon stick
2–3 dried lavender heads
4 firm pears, peeled, stalk attached

1 Heat the honey and lemon juice in a heavy pan until the honey has dissolved. Add the water, saffron threads, cinnamon stick and the flowers from 1–2 lavender heads. Bring to the boil, reduce the heat, then simmer for 5 minutes.

2 Add the whole pears to the pan and simmer gently for 20 minutes until they are tender. Leave to cool in the syrup and serve at room temperature, decorated with a few lavender flowers.

Energy 283Kcal/1,207kJ; **Protein** 0.8g; **Carbohydrate** 74.3g, of which sugars 74.3g; **Fat** 0.2g, of which saturates 0g; **Cholesterol** 0mg; **Calcium** 38mg; **Fibre** 3.3g; **Sodium** 10mg.

Ricotta honey cakes with fruit sauce
INGREDIENTS
Serves 4

250g/9oz/generous 1 cup ricotta cheese
2 egg whites
60ml/4 tbsp scented honey, plus extra to taste
450g/1lb/4 cups mixed fresh or frozen fruit, such as strawberries, raspberries or cherries

1 Preheat the oven to 180°C/350°F/ Gas 4. Beat the ricotta with the egg whites and honey until smooth. Grease four ramekins. Spoon in the mixture and level the tops. Bake for 20 minutes.

2 For the fruit sauce, reserve some fruit for decoration, put the rest in a pan, with water if the fruit is fresh, and heat until soft. Cool slightly and remove any stones (pits). Press through a sieve, and sweeten with honey. Serve the sauce, warm or cold, with the cakes. Decorate with the reserved berries.

Energy 176Kcal/741kJ; **Protein** 8g; **Carbohydrate** 21g, of which sugars 21g; **Fat** 7g, of which saturates 4g; **Cholesterol** 31mg; **Calcium** 173mg; **Fibre** 1.4g; **Sodium** 100mg.

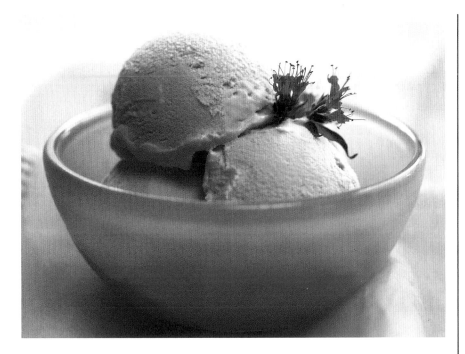

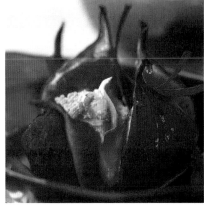

Crème fraîche and honey ice

This delicately flavoured vanilla ice cream is delicious served with hot apple pie.

INGREDIENTS

Serves 4

4 egg yolks
60ml/4 tbsp clear flower honey
5ml/1 tsp cornflour (cornstarch)
300ml/½ pint/1¼ cups milk
7.5ml/1½ tsp natural vanilla extract
250g/9oz/generous 1 cup crème fraîche
nasturtium or herb flowers, to decorate

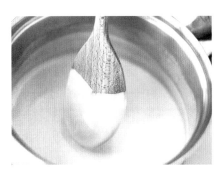

1 Whisk the egg yolks, honey and cornflour in a bowl until thick and foamy. Bring the milk to the boil, then pour on to the yolk mixture, whisking.

Energy 386Kcal/1602kJ; **Protein** 6.9g; **Carbohydrate** 16.5g, of which sugars 16.3g; **Fat** 33g, of which saturates 19.5g; **Cholesterol** 277mg; **Calcium** 151mg; **Fibre** 0g; **Sodium** 57mg.

2 Return the mixture to the pan and cook over low heat, stirring all the time until the custard thickens and is smooth. Pour it back into the bowl, then set aside until cool.

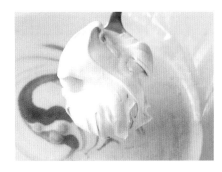

3 Stir in the vanilla extract and crème fraîche. Pour into a plastic tub or similar freezerproof container. Freeze for about 6 hours or until firm enough to scoop, beating once or twice with a fork or in a food processor to break up the ice crystals.

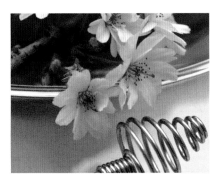

Fresh figs baked with honey

Baking fruit with honey is an ancient cooking method.

INGREDIENTS

Serves 4

12 ripe figs
30ml/2 tbsp sugar
3–4 cinnamon sticks
45–60ml/3–4 tbsp clear honey
225g/8oz/1 cup natural (plain) yogurt

1 Preheat the oven to 200°C/400°F/ Gas 6. Wash the figs and pat dry with kitchen paper. Cut a deep cross from the top of each fig to the bottom, keeping the skin at the bottom intact. Fan each fig out to look like a flower, then place upright in a baking tin (pan).

2 Sprinkle the sugar over each fig flower, tuck in the cinnamon sticks and drizzle with the honey. Bake for about 15–20 minutes, until the sugar is slightly caramelized but the honey and figs are still moist. Check to make sure they are not browning too much and if they are, cover them with baking foil for the rest of the cooking time.

3 Remove the cinnamon sticks before serving the figs. Eat warm with yogurt.

Energy 198Kcal/845kJ; **Protein** 2.3g; **Carbohydrate** 48.2g, of which sugars 48.2g; **Fat** 1g, of which saturates 0g; **Cholesterol** 0mg; **Calcium** 155mg; **Fibre** 4.5g; **Sodium** 39mg.

HONEY IN BAKING

Honey particularly lends itself to aromatically spiced cakes and cookies and is a favourite in any sweet bars and buns. Honey attracts moisture so that baked goods stay moist and fresh.

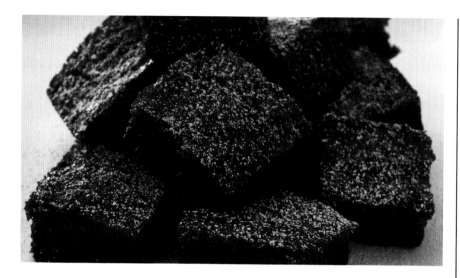

Spicy honey cake
INGREDIENTS

Serves 8

175g/6oz/1½ cups plain (all-purpose) flour

75g/3oz/⅓ cup caster (superfine) sugar

2.5ml/½ tsp ground ginger

2.5–5ml/½–1 tsp ground cinnamon

5ml/1 tsp mixed (apple pie) spice

5ml/1 tsp bicarbonate of soda
 (baking soda)

225g/8oz/1 cup clear honey

60ml/4 tbsp vegetable or olive oil

grated rind of 1 orange

2 eggs

75ml/5 tbsp orange juice

10ml/2 tsp chopped fresh root ginger

1 Preheat the oven to 180°C/350°F/ Gas 4. Line a rectangular baking tin (pan), measuring 25 x 20 x 5cm/ 10 x 8 x 2in, with a sheet of baking parchment. In a large mixing bowl, stir together the flour, sugar, ginger, cinnamon, mixed spice and bicarbonate of soda.

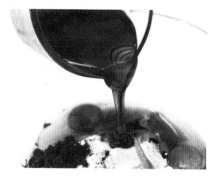

2 Make a well in the centre of the flour mixture and pour in the honey, oil, orange rind and eggs. Beat until smooth, then add the orange juice and ginger.

3 Pour the cake mixture into the prepared tin, then bake for about 50 minutes, or until firm to the touch.

4 Leave the cake to cool in the tin, then turn out and wrap tightly in foil. Store at room temperature for 2–3 days before serving to allow the flavours of the cake to mature.

Energy 152Kcal/640kJ; **Protein** 1.9g; **Carbohydrate** 23.6g, of which sugars 13g; **Fat** 6.3g, of which saturates 3.8g; **Cholesterol** 26mg; **Calcium** 30mg; **Fibre** 0.4g; **Sodium** 49mg.

Honey cookies
INGREDIENTS

Makes 20

2.5ml/½ tsp bicarbonate of soda
 (baking soda)

grated rind and juice of 1 large orange

150ml/¼ pint/⅔ cup extra virgin olive oil

75g/3oz/6 tbsp caster (superfine) sugar

60ml/4 tbsp brandy

7.5ml/1½ tsp ground cinnamon

400g/14oz/3½ cups self-raising (self-rising)
 flour, sifted with a pinch of salt

225g/8oz/1 cup clear honey

115g/4oz/½ cup caster (superfine) sugar

115g/4oz/1 cup walnuts, chopped,
 to decorate

1 Mix the bicarbonate of soda and orange juice. Beat the oil with the sugar, add the brandy and cinnamon, then add to the orange juice. Add the flour and salt into the mixture, then the orange rind, and knead for 10 minutes.

2 Preheat the oven to 180°C/350°F/ Gas 4. Flour your hands and shape small pieces of dough into ovals and place on baking sheets. Flatten the cookies a little, then bake for 25 minutes. Cool.

3 Bring the honey, sugar and 150ml/ ¼ pint/⅔ cup water to the boil, skim, then simmer for 5 minutes. Immerse the cookies in the syrup for 2 minutes. Sprinkle with the walnuts.

Energy 118Kcal/495kJ; **Protein** 1.3g; **Carbohydrate** 17.3g, of which sugars 10.1g; **Fat 5.3**g, of which saturates 3.2g; **Cholesterol** 26mg; **Calcium** 21mg; **Fibre** 0.3g; **Sodium** 39mg.

Honey and walnut bars
INGREDIENTS

Makes 12–14

175g/6oz/1½ cups plain (all-purpose) flour

30ml/2 tbsp icing (confectioners')
  sugar, sifted

115g/4oz/½ cup unsalted (sweet)
  butter, diced

For the topping

300g/11oz/scant 3 cups walnut halves

2 eggs, beaten

50g/2oz/¼ cup unsalted (sweet)
  butter, melted

50g/2oz/¼ cup light muscovado
  (brown) sugar

90ml/6 tbsp dark clear honey

30ml/2 tbsp single (light) cream

1 Preheat the oven to 190°C/375°F/Gas 5. Grease a 28 x 18cm/11 x 7in tin (pan).

2 Put the flour, icing sugar and butter in a food processor and process until the mixture forms crumbs. Using the pulse button, add 15–30ml/1–2 tbsp water – enough to make a firm dough.

3 Roll the dough out and line the base and sides of the tin. Trim and fold the top edge inwards.

4 Prick the base, line with foil and baking beans and bake blind for 10 minutes. Remove the foil and beans. Return to the oven for 5 minutes, until cooked but not browned. Reduce the temperature to 180°C/350°F/Gas 4.

5 For the topping, sprinkle the nuts over the base. Whisk the remaining ingredients. Pour over the walnuts and bake for 25 minutes. Leave to cool.

Energy: 333Kcal/1,386kJ; **Protein** 5.4g; **Carbohydrate** 21.4g, of which sugars 11.7g; **Fat** 25.7g, of which saturates 7.8g; **Cholesterol** 53mg; **Calcium** 49mg; **Fibre** 1.1g; **Sodium** 85mg.

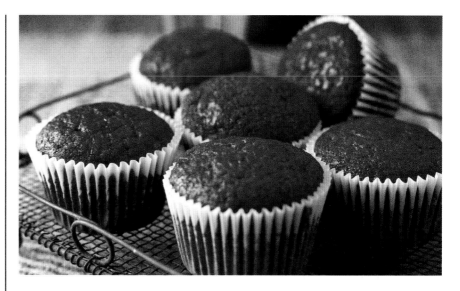

Honey and spice cakes
INGREDIENTS

Makes 18

250g/9oz/2 cups plain (all-purpose) flour

5ml/1 tsp ground cinnamon

5ml/1 tsp bicarbonate of soda (baking soda)

125g/4½oz/½ cup butter, softened

125g/4½oz/½ cup soft brown sugar

1 large (US extra large) egg, separated

125g/4½oz clear honey

about 60ml/4 tbsp milk

caster (superfine) sugar, for sprinkling

1 Preheat the oven to 200°C/400°F/Gas 6. Lightly butter a bun tin (pan) or line the bun tin with paper cases.

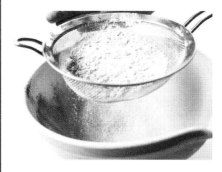

2 Sift the flour into a large mixing bowl with the cinnamon and the bicarbonate of soda.

3 Beat the butter with the sugar until light and fluffy. Beat in the egg yolk, then gradually add the honey.

4 With a large metal spoon and a cutting action, fold in the flour mixture plus sufficient milk to make a soft mixture that will just drop off the spoon.

5 In a separate bowl, whisk the egg white until stiff peaks form. With a large metal spoon, using a figure-of-eight movement, fold the egg white into the cake mixture.

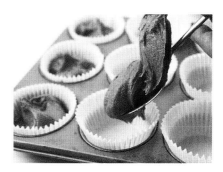

6 Divide the mixture among the paper cases or distribute the mixture in the prepared tin. Put into the hot oven and cook for 15–20 minutes or until risen, firm and springy to the touch and golden brown.

7 Sprinkle the tops of the buns lightly with caster sugar, then leave to cool completely on a wire rack.

Energy 152Kcal/639kJ; **Protein** 1.9g; **Carbohydrate** 23.6g, of which sugars 13g; **Fat** 6.3g, of which saturates 3.8g; **Cholesterol** 26mg; **Calcium** 30mg; **Fibre** 0.4g; **Sodium** 49mg.

HONEY IN DRESSINGS, RELISHES AND DIPS

Honey is surprisingly delicious in salad dressings, adding a sweet touch that complements many ingredients. Dips and relishes also benefit from the addition of honey.

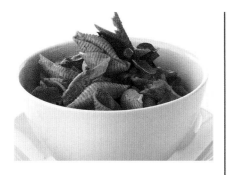

Honey and mustard dressing

This tangy dressing gives a kick to a tuna, pasta and corn salad.

In a bowl, mix 60ml/4 tbsp extra virgin olive oil, 15ml/1 tbsp balsamic vinegar, 5ml/1 tsp red wine vinegar, and 5ml/1 tsp Dijon mustard with 10ml/2 tsp clear honey. Add to the salad and toss well to mix.

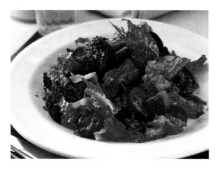

Honey and herb dressing

Mixed herbs, honey, oil and lemon are a perfect foil for a spicy sausage salad.

Mix 30ml/2 tbsp lemon juice, 15ml/1 tbsp clear honey, 90ml/6 tbsp olive oil, 10ml/2 tsp French mustard, 30ml/2 tbsp chopped fresh herbs, such as coriander (cilantro), chives and parsley. Pour over the salad.

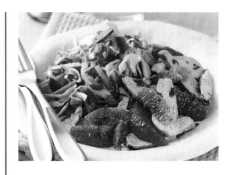

Honey and citrus dressing

Orange rind and juice, honey and oil make a light, zesty dressing for chicken.

To 15ml/1 tbsp honey, add the juice and grated rind of 1 orange, segments from 2 limes, 30ml/2 tbsp chopped tarragon and 60ml/4 tbsp olive oil. Mix thoroughly, season to taste and spoon over a chicken salad.

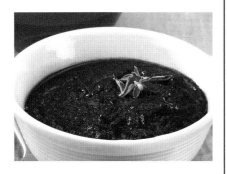

Honey and chipotle relish

This smoky-flavoured relish is great in sandwiches or just served on its own.

Drain 400g/14oz can tomatoes. Discard the juice. In a blender or food processor, mix the tomatoes, 5 chipotle chillies, 3 garlic cloves, 60ml/4 tbsp clear honey, 5ml/1 tsp dried oregano, 5ml/1 tsp American mustard and 150ml/¼ pint/²⁄₃ cup red wine. Process until smooth. Serve with grilled (broiled) or barbecued meats.

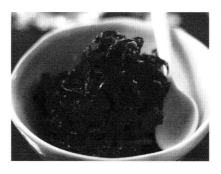

Honey, carrot and almond relish

This honeyed relish is a perfect accompaniment to grilled meat.

In a pan, mix 15ml/1 tbsp ground coriander with 500g/1¼lb grated carrots, 50g/2oz shredded root ginger, juice and grated rind of 1 lemon, and 30ml/2 tbsp clear honey with 120ml/4fl oz/½ cup wine vinegar. Bring to the boil, then simmer for 30 minutes until the mixure has thickened, stirring often. Add 50g/2oz/½ cup flaked almonds and serve.

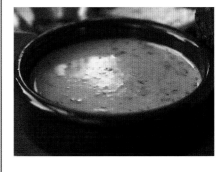

Honey and sesame dip

Sesame, lemon and honey combine with mint to make a sweet and tangy dip.

Beat 15ml/3 tbsp light sesame paste with the juice of 1 lemon. Add 30ml/2 tbsp clear honey and 5–10ml/1–2 tsp dried mint and beat again until the mixture is thick and creamy. Spoon into a small dish and serve at room temperature with lemon wedges for squeezing. This dip is good served with chunks of crusty fresh bread or toasted pitta bread.

HONEY IN MARINADES AND GLAZES

Honey is excellent in savoury dishes, especially in marinades or glazes, when it adds a unique flavour and glossy stickiness to roasted or barbecued meat, poultry and even fruits.

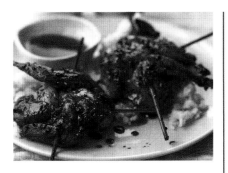

Honey and garlic marinade
Garlic, honey and mushroom soy sauce make a delicious marinade for quails.

In a bowl, beat 150ml/¼ pint/⅔ cup mushroom soy sauce with 45ml/3 tbsp honey. Stir in 8 crushed garlic cloves, 15ml/1 tbsp crushed black peppercorns and 30ml/2 tbsp sesame oil.

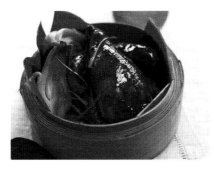

Honey and orange marinade
A spicy honey and citrus coating ensures that poultry is moist and succulent.

Combine the juice and grated rind of 2 oranges, 2 crushed garlic cloves, 15ml/1 tbsp chopped root ginger, 45ml/3 tbsp soy sauce, 75ml/5 tbsp honey and 2–3 star anise with 30ml/2 tbsp rice wine.

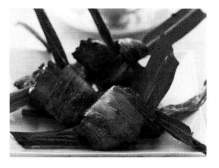

Honey and ginger marinade
Ginger, sour plum sauce and honey are natural partners in this tasty marinade.

Grind 6 chopped shallots, 4 chopped garlic cloves and 25g/1oz root ginger to a smooth paste. Beat in 30ml/2 tbsp honey, 30ml/ 2 tbsp each tomato ketchup and sour plum sauce and 15ml/1 tbsp sesame oil.

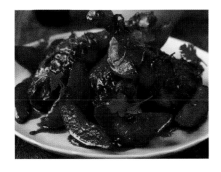

Honey and spice glaze
Ginger, cinnamon and honey add a fruity, spicy flavour to duck.

Melt 30ml/2 tbsp butter in a pan. Stir in 25g/1oz peeled and grated fresh root ginger and cook for about 1 minute. Add 10ml/ 2 tsp ground cinnamon, 30ml/2 tbsp clear honey and the juice of 1 lemon. Add 30–45ml/2–3 tbsp water and stir until it bubbles. Simmer until the glaze is reduced and shiny, then pour over roasted meat.

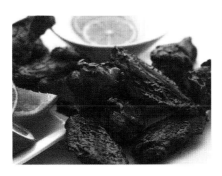

Honey and mustard glaze
When mixed with a tangy mustard, honey peps up chicken wings or legs.

In a small bowl, mix 60ml/4 tbsp clear honey, with 60ml/4 tbsp wholegrain mustard. Beat well and season with salt and ground black pepper to taste. Brush the mixture over chicken portions before grilling (broiling) or barbecuing. Renew the glaze towards the end of the cooking time and make sure that the glaze does not burn.

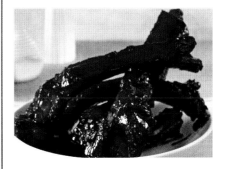

Honey and soy glaze
Mixed with soy sauce, honey adds a sticky sweet and sour flavour to ribs.

Mix together 75ml/5 tbsp clear honey with 75ml/5 tbsp light soy sauce. Pour or brush over pork spare ribs, turning them several times to ensure they are thoroughly coated. Bake the ribs for 30 minutes at 190°C/ 375°F/Gas 5, then increase the oven temperature to 220°C/425°F/Gas 7 until there is a thick, sticky glaze on the ribs.

INDEX

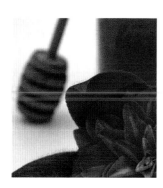
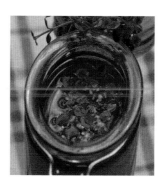
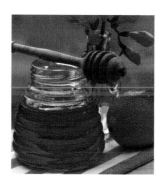
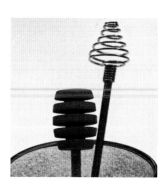

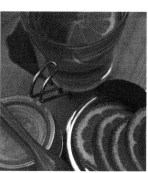
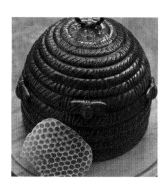
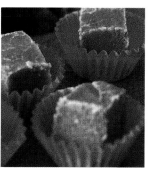
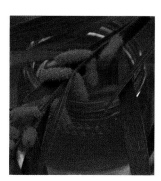

DISCARD

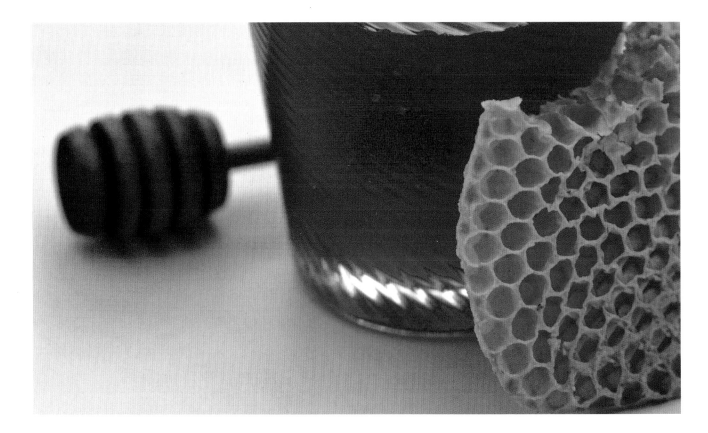

Acknowledgements

The author and publishers would like to thank the following individuals and companies for their valuable contributions to this book:

Beekeeper Laurie Wiseman for sharing his expertise.

Rowse Honey Limited for supplying samples from their extensive range of honeys for taste tests and for photography.

The Hive Honey Shop, the largest supplier of English honey and honeybee-related products in the UK, for supplying honey products and artifacts.

The Hive Honey Shop
93 Northcote Road,
London SW11 6PL
Tel. 020 7924 6233
www.thehivehoneyshop.co.uk

Websites and reading

Useful websites
www.honeyassociation.com
www.nhb.org
www.rowsehoney.co.uk

Further reading
Bishop, Holley, *Robbing the Bees* (Simon & Schuster, London, 2005)
Honey, a Book of Recipes (Lorenz Books, London, 1997)
Monk Kidd, Sue, *The Secret Life of Bees* (Headline Book Publishing Ltd, London, 2002)

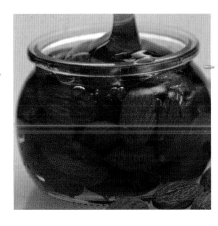

Picture credits

The publisher would like to thank the following picture libraries for the use of their pictures in the book. Every effort has been made to acknowledge the pictures properly.

l=left, r=right, t=top, b=bottom, bl=bottom left, br=bottom right, m=middle, tr=top right.

Art Archive: 11br; 34.
Bridgeman Art Library: 10, 16.
Corbis: 6m; 11tl; 12t, 12bl &12br; 14; 15b; 17tr; 18t; 19bl; 20bl & 20tr; 21br; 35r; 63tl.
Felicity Forster: 8, 15tr.
NHPA: 17bl; 18bl.
Nature Picture Library: 13bl; 30tr.
Science Photo Library: 13r.